Mary Lou Gryzba

Psalm 9:1-2

ISBN: 978-0-692-25654-1

Unless otherwise indicated, Scripture quotations are taken from The
Holy Bible, New Living Translation®, © 1996, 2004, 2007, 2013 by
Tyndale House Foundation. Used by permission of Tyndale House
Publishers Inc., Carol Stream, Illinois 60188. All rights reserved.

Scripture quotations taken from the Amplified® Bible. © 1954,
1958, 1962, 1964, 1965, 1987 by The Lockman Foundation. Used by
permission. Lockman.org

Used by permission. Jesus Calling, Sarah Young, 2004, 2011, Thomas
Nelson. Nashville, Tennessee. All rights reserved.

Contents

Preface   7

One | Change in a Day   13

Two | Learning a New Routine   29

Three | Branching Out and Being Stretched   51

Four | A Longer Journey   73

Five | Long Hot July   95

Six | Learning More and Moving Past Me   139

Seven | "I Want My Mommy"   153

Eight | Seeing Him In Spite of Me   173

Nine | The Aftermath   189

Ten | The Lord Prepares   203

Epilogue   229

Hidden Crosses   234

Acknowledgements   235

Preface

Throughout our lives God gives us new experiences that challenge and stretch our faith and also teaches us how much we really do need Him. I remember when my first baby was born. Since I'd never been a mother, I relied on others who'd made the journey, which was very helpful and encouraging...but at the end of the day it was me and God, working through my new, tender emotions. Even reading the famous *What to Expect When You're Expecting* was helpful and gave me a "heads up" on what was coming month to month. But honestly, there's no amount of information or testimonies that can really prepare you for

being a mom...you just learn as you go through the experience.

The same is true when caring for an elderly parent. You
would think that if you've know someone all your life, taking care of them would be a piece of cake. Just as brand
new emotions surface as a new mother, so they surface as a
caregiver. And even though the encouragement and testimonies from other caregivers keeps you moving forward
with hope, you still have to go through the experience yourself, hitting every emotional and physical challenge head on!
And even though you stand firm on the faith, the promises
and the power of the Lord Jesus Christ, you still have to go
THROUGH the storm. The "rubber meets the road" in your
Christian walk when you take what you know by faith in
your head and heart and apply it in your storm.

I wrote this book with the simple intent to share. For six
months I cared for my parents and boy, did I learn a lot...in
fact, I'm still growing. I humbly admit I'm not an expert on
the art of taking care of an elderly parent. I only have one
thing, and that's my testimony. It's just my story, plain and
simple. I would love to say that my story is a triumphant
one with me being the heroine and mighty princess warrior.
Instead, it's a story of how to get through something with
difficulty as you hang on to an amazing, loving God.

In ministry at church, I teach, share and become completely transparent with the college age group. These guys

and girls have no interest in surface feelings and fluff. They want to know the real deal. They want to know the raw emotions of your testimony and life experiences. This is the approach I took in this book. So many times we walk out our Christian lives with a "buck up" and "suck it up" attitude to save face and appear to have it together, when on the inside we're crying out to God and hoping maybe He will send someone who will say, "I understand those deep emotional feelings." I know that the caregiving experiences of others may be far more heartbreaking and challenging than mine, yet I suspect some of the emotions are similar. Throughout my experience with my daddy, I developed a new respect and awareness for caregivers that quite frankly, you just never truly are aware of until you join that club yourself.

Throughout the book I quote small passages on various days from my devotional, *Jesus Calling* by Sarah Young. These particular days really ministered to me and always surprised and comforted me in God's perfect timing. I also inserted the exact entries that I wrote from my personal journal. I hope and pray this story of my experience brings laughter, tears and encouragement to other caregivers. I especially hope that by reading this book the feelings of guilt, shame and disappointment will wash away from the caregiver who is struggling with feelings they never anticipated feeling. Finding someone who understands those feelings exposes the lie that says, "You are alone." Well, you are NOT alone. While I can't do one thing to change a caregiver's unexpected journey, my prayer is that I can hopefully help them with the emotional part of that journey.

Also, never underestimate how God answers prayers or encourages your heart. Trust Him to be God and never put boundaries on Him. Yes, He uses His Word and people. But stretch your faith and believe He'll use the unexpected. Like redbirds.

Blessings,
Mary Jo Graham

CHAPTER ONE

Change in a Day

I'll never forget June 6, 2012. My 18-year-old daughter, Mary Lee, and I were shopping in Franklin, Tennessee and enjoying the beautiful day. Some shopping days are meant for shopping, but other shopping days are meant for just being together. This was a day for mother and daughter to just simply be together. Because the weather was so nice, I thought walking in and out of shops on the town square would be fun, especially with a latte in hand. There was one particular store I wanted to go in because I knew they would have the perfect gift for a friend of mine. She had just lost her husband a couple weeks earlier and I

had not bought her a gift, just to say "I'm thinking about
you." As we pulled into the parking lot Mary Lee looked
at her cell phone and said, "Daddy is trying to call you." I
pulled the car into park and turned the engine off, then immediately called my husband, Jeff. His first words were,
"Mary Jo, have you talked to your mother?" I said, "No,
why?" He said, "She's had an accident and they're taking
her to the emergency room." This was such a strange thing
for me to hear. My mother? An accident?

You have to understand, my 73-year-old mother is amazing. She doesn't look her age; she's very intelligent, has tons
of energy and for the past five plus years has been the sole
caregiver for my 83-year-old daddy. My mother is physically strong and her hobby is working in her yard, planting
flowers, plants and shrubs. Just give her a mound of dirt
and she is happy. She also volunteers at the hospital, helps
on church projects and quite frankly, doesn't have a selfish
bone in her body. She takes care of all of her and Daddy's
personal finances, has great computer skills and even knows
how to text! She is a retired executive secretary and is incredibly organized and detailed, yet never high-minded or
unteachable. So to say that my mother, Rhoda Gunter, had
an accident just didn't compute in my thinking. I got off the
phone with Jeff and called my mother's cell phone.

To my surprise she answered and out of her mouth
came, "Honey, I'm so sorry. I was trying to cut a limb off the

tree and my saw pulled me off the ladder."

"Are you OK?"

"Well, my legs hurt and the ambulance is here."

"Is Daddy OK? Is somebody with him?"

"Yes, I think one of the neighbors is in the house now telling him I fell. He's going to be so upset. He has always told me, "Mama, please don't climb or do anything foolish... if you hurt yourself, then where would I be?"

"Mama, I'm leaving Franklin now and I'm on my way to the emergency room...I'll meet you there...I love you...it's going to be OK."

I could hear commotion in the background and her say again before she hung up, "Honey, I'm so so sorry."

• • • •

For the past five years I've been an educational assistant at a middle school. After being a stay-at-home mom for 14 years with my family, I was really enjoying working again. My job was working in the library. Having a corporate and personnel background didn't qualify me to be a library assistant, and when a friend told me about the job, I hesitated thinking, "A librarian? This is not even in my top 100 job possibilities." But from the first day I started, I fell in love with the librarian, Christine, and I loved the job. Seeing the middle school kids, doing computer work, working on administrative projects and discovering a love for middle school books made going into work pure joy. And when you work in the school system you become like a kid again. You look forward to holiday breaks, snow days and especially the last day of school. Knowing that nine weeks of summer was before me was a huge adrenaline rush! So for five years I never dreaded going into work. I also enjoyed the time off, knowing I'd be starting a new school year again.

Sometime around the beginning of 2012, the Lord began speaking to my heart. This was nothing audible, but I had a strong feeling that this was going to be my last year at the middle school. So over the next several months I started praying about what He wanted me to do. You see, I believe God found me this job and planted me there for a purpose. So if He was saying it was time to go, then I knew He had a plan and another job waiting for me. And if He knew I'd totally enjoy being a librarian, then I could trust Him to find me the next job, wherever it was. I decided I'd just share with a few friends so they would pray too. After all, I did want to make sure I was hearing from God because this was such a great job. I even asked God if I needed to get a resume together or start looking. Over the remaining months of school, every time I would ask He replied in my heart with the same answer, *"Just Wait."*

One day Christine walked up behind me at my desk, put her hands on my shoulder and whispered in my ear, "You're not coming back next year, are you?"

Confirmation? Maybe. I told her, "Well, I don't know. I'm not looking for another job...I just don't know. But as soon as I do, you'll be the first to know. "

• • • •

Driving from Franklin back to my home in Murfrees-boro, which is only a thirty minute drive, seemed like a life-time. Mary Lee and I prayed out loud for Mama and asked God to just go ahead and heal her legs. But in my heart I knew there was going to be more than just a quick check sending her back home. When I got to the house to drop Mary Lee off, I figured I'd better grab a change of clothes too. In fact, as I mindlessly packed, I threw in toiletries and a few extra clothes, as well as my Bible and *Jesus Calling* devotional by Sarah Young. I was thankful that when the mind is blank the body knows what to do. I felt like I was on auto pilot. Jeff was out of town, so we talked off and on while I hurried to get to my parents' house in Shelbyville. He didn't ask me a lot of questions. I think he knew this situation could be serious. Plus, when I'm in task mode, like packing, I'm probably not listening anyway. I told him I'd call him as soon as I knew something. The forty-five minute drive from my house to Shelbyville was equally long. I honestly felt like I was driving backwards. My mind was racing on who to call and what to do. First, I called the neighbor to check on Daddy. He said he was fine and that he could stay with him

until I got there. So I decided to go straight to the emergency room and see for myself how bad this fall was.

My next call during the drive was to my dad's sister,
Aunt Mary, who lived in Nashville. In the past she had
stayed with Daddy if Mama was out of town, but that was
years ago. As I told her what happened and asked if she
could stay with Daddy, she so gently reminded me that
she was also 73 years old and if "Brother" fell there was no
way she could help. Being the incredible trooper she is, she
graciously said she would do whatever I needed her to do.
But at that moment, I knew instantly that she wouldn't be
spending the night...I would. Then I remembered that I had
packed clothes. Deep down I guess I already knew. I told
her that I needed to think a minute and I'd call her back. But
I knew. I knew it was me. I knew that my life was going to
change. I knew I'd need more clothes. I knew this was going to be longer than a few days. And then it dawned on me
what God had spoken in my heart for months..."*Just Wait.*"

"Oh, dear Lord...this is why I'm not going back to school
in the fall isn't it?" I wasn't sure whether to cry, to panic
or to just pray. Frankly, I was too scared to think or plan. I
knew my mother needed me and that was where I would
focus...at least for the time being.

As I rushed into the hospital emergency room I made eye
contact with the first employee I saw. She was in the admitting area, so I knew she'd help. "I'm Rhoda Gunter's daugh-

ter and …." Before I could finish she pushed a button that opened two double doors.

"Go down the hall and to the left. The nurses will show you where she is," she graciously replied. As I swiftly walked down the hall, I continued to pray softly, "Lord, heal her." I walked up to the nurses' station and asked where Mama was. She just pointed, so I made a 180-degree turn, and lying in a corner room was my mama. Linda, her neighbor across the street, sat beside her. As I walked toward her, she looked up and saw me then began to cry and repeat what she had said over the phone earlier, "Honey, I'm so sorry." My mother is so confident and assured, but the look on her face was filled with guilt and regret. She knew, just as I knew, our lives and routine were about to change.

"Mama, it's going to be OK," I said, as I leaned over to kiss her cheek. "Are you hurting?" She was sort of sitting up with her legs straight out. They weren't cut or bruised or anything.

"Well, they hurt pretty bad and I can't seem to move them," she said. I glanced at Linda, and she just shook her head as if to say, "This isn't good."

After the x-rays were taken the doctor came to talk with us. They referred to the results as fractures and said that the "fracture" in the right leg was worse than the left. I was thinking, "OK…fracture. Maybe that's not too bad. Maybe that's like something you wrap up like a sprain and in a few weeks it's healed." Having never had a "fracture," I wasn't sure.

I finally just point blank asked the nurse, "What do the x-rays really mean?"

"Well, both of your mother's legs are broken. Because osteoporosis is in both knees, the tibia bones broke into the knees and shattered them. In fact, the right is worse because it broke in two places."

These breaks were so bad that they were considered a trauma break, which required a specialized trauma doctor. As this was being explained to my mother, she had a look of complete disbelief on her face. She was having "trauma" of the heart and mind as well as in her legs. She was so in shock that this was happening to her.

Since Shelbyville didn't have a "trauma doctor" the ER doctor called Williamson Medical Center in Franklin. They agreed to have her transported there. As they prepared for her to go in the ambulance, I knew I wouldn't be making this trip. I called Aunt Mary and told her I needed her to meet Mama at the hospital and that I would go home to be with Daddy.

Leaving Mama was hard. She cried so much. She continued to apologize and ask for forgiveness. She was a mess. I told her it was going to be OK and that Daddy would be fine.

When I left the ER, I walked to the car, got in and proceeded to break down and cry. Now I'm a pretty capable, independent woman, but at this moment I felt like a helpless little girl. "Oh God, I'm so scared! Please help me! I don't know what to do with Daddy!" I felt so helpless and terrified over so many unknowns. I needed major prayer. Fortunately, God has blessed my life with some pretty amazing godly girlfriends. These are the kind of women that will get in the trenches with you and cover you with prayer. I sent out a mass text to about 12 of these friends. Here's the great thing about these women: I didn't have to go into a ton of details. I knew they would go straight to God in prayer and He would show them how to pray. The Body of Christ is so incredible. Just pushing the Send button on my cell phone brought a portion of peace I needed in order to keep moving. I decided as I drove to Mama and Daddy's house that I needed to be positive and strong for Daddy. One thing I knew was my daddy, Billy Gunter, was a champion worrier. No matter what, I had to stay positive.

• • • •

For as long as I can remember my daddy has called my mother, "Mama." Don't you love the way older couples call each other "Mama" and "Daddy"? Now my mother is proper, so she only calls him Billy, but she was always "Mama." Sometimes my mother would correct him and say, "Billy, I am not your mama. Don't call me 'Mama!' He

would always reply, "How about I call you 'Big Mama!'"
Then he'd laugh and laugh. In any relationship you have
a straight man and well, the one who thinks everything is
funny. That's my dad. He always likes a good laugh and
never has a serious bone in his body, yet the flip side is that
he is a habitual worrier--the kind where he concocts things
in his head and lets the worry just build and build until it's
so out of range it's hard to pull it down with any kind of
logic or reasoning. My mother on the other hand is very
positive and likes to talk things through. She is open to others' opinions; and if she doesn't agree she's perfectly content
that it's OK that there are two opinions.

My daddy...where do I start? Daddy was always the
cut-up, picker, agitator, sociable, routine guy. He was
retired from the post office and everybody in town knew
him. For forty plus years my daddy always did the grocery
shopping. Every Saturday morning since I can remember he
would get up and go to the grocery store. To him it wasn't
primarily about the groceries. This was a social outing. He
would leave around 9:00am and sometimes wouldn't come
back until lunchtime. So many newcomers to Shelbyville
would say that Billy Gunter was the first person they met,
either at Kroger or the post office. Their stories were the
same as to how he not only introduced himself first, but
then he would also introduce someone else to them. He was
like an ambassador! Oh, and I wish you could have seen

him work a funeral!   Because he grew up in Shelbyville and knew everyone in town he had some kind of connection with most everyone who died too! He could make the grieving families smile or sometimes laugh by telling an old story about their loved one. Then after paying his respects he'd proceed to introducing people to each other. But as lovable and funny as my daddy was, well, we all have flaws. And my daddy had a quick temper and was a negative worrier, and I could tell the older he got the more negative he could be. Over the past several years my daddy had battled with diabetes, heart by-pass surgery, a shunt in his head (from fluid on the brain), Meniere's, no circulation in his legs and early stages of dementia. Yes, he could be so negative and irritable at times; but by the grace of God, the silly humor remained in tack.

• • • •

"How's Mama?" were my daddy's first words when he saw me walk in the door. So how do you sugar-coat this accident? How do you make two broken legs sound not so bad? And how on earth do you tell him that his caregiver will be taking a leave of absence...and that there's a new rookie on the job!

"Well Daddy, it's not good. Mama has 'fractured' (I thought it sounded better and a little vague) her legs, so she's going to have to have surgery. But I'm going to stay

with you as long as I need to, and it's going to be OK."
There, that sounded good. After all, my mother is strong.
Combine that with the healing power of Almighty God and I
figure this set-up won't last too long.

"Is she OK?" Hmm, I thought I just answered that, but
he was concerned about her emotional state too.

"She is out of it right now. They've taken her to Williamson Medical Center in Franklin, and Aunt Mary is going to
meet her there."

Neighbor Linda's husband, Lavon, had been sitting in
the den with Daddy when I walked in the house. He decided it was best to say his goodbyes and go home. I thanked
him for all his help and told him I'd be in touch. Now it was
just me and Daddy. As I sat down on the sofa across from
Daddy it flashed through my mind that I didn't have a clue
what his needs were. I knew Daddy had been using a walker for quite a while, but that's about it. My mind was racing
as I thought about where I'd sleep, how to cook for him and
oh yes, how to pay the bills! But all of this would come soon
enough. For right now I needed to just sit down and talk to
him…and to let him talk.

"Jo,…" My daddy has always called me Jo. "Jo, I have
told her over and over, 'Please don't climb.' But your mama
doesn't listen. She's going to do whatever she wants to do.
Now look at this mess."

"Well, we'll know more in a little bit." I tried so hard to

keep the seriousness away from his thinking, but this was pretty much impossible.

Shortly after this my mother called. Thank goodness for cell phones! She said, "Well, there's not a trauma doctor that can do this kind of surgery at Williamson Medical Center. They said I'll be transported to Vanderbilt Medical Hospital as soon as they have a room available." Mama was still mentally sound and didn't sound like she was in shock or anything. She did say her legs were hurting and the pain level was pretty bad. For Mama to say it's painful means it's excruciating. She has a very high pain tolerance. Of course, again throughout the details of her explaining what was next, my sweet mother continued to apologize and verbally beat herself up. "Why did I think that tree limb had to come down? Why didn't I just wait and call someone to do it? Honey, I'm so sorry. I've messed up your summer and your being with Mary Lee. Please tell Jeff I am so sorry." The guilt just continued to flow like a running faucet as she would cry and cry.

I have to honestly say I never once thought, "Mother, what were you thinking!?" I was actually thinking that if bets had been made on whether or not my mother could successfully cut down the tree limb, I would have bet on my mother every time! In fact, there was a hint of pride welling up in me that said, "My 73-year-old mother cuts down tree limbs." It sounds crazy but I was proud of her.

As Mother traveled to Vanderbilt Hospital, my aunt went as well, and my mother's niece called to say she would be there too. I felt at peace knowing that both of these two competent women could keep me informed.

"Daddy, Mama has to go to Vanderbilt so the right doctor can do the surgery. She's on her way now."

"VANDERBILT! How bad is this?"

"It's considered a trauma break so it has to be the right doctor who has experience."

Over the course of the next few hours I felt like Daddy and I were going around the same mountain of questions and answers. I could feel and hear the worry rising. But I knew all I could do was continue to answer the questions as respectfully and honestly as I could, knowing that no answer would really help.

CHAPTER TWO

Learning a New Routine

T hinking about the first couple of days of caring for Daddy is kind of fuzzy to me now. I do recall reading the June 7th in <u>Jesus Calling</u>. A portion of it read,

> "Who is in charge of your life? If it is you, then you
> have good reason to worry. But if it is I, then worry is
> both unnecessary and counterproductive."

It is amazing how a devotional can so clearly speak to your circumstances. Over the next several months this little devotional proved to line up so closely with my life, my emotions, and my unfamiliar journey.

When caring for an elderly parent you tend to switch over to a moment-to-moment mentality and just do what you need to do. I can't remember enough to describe in detail, or the order of sequence, but I learned over the next 48 hours the needs of my daddy. I learned that Daddy wore adult disposable underwear with big maxi pads in them. He called them "pretends" instead because he said you pretend you're peeing on your own. I learned that he used a urinal when he couldn't make it to the bathroom with the walker. So my mother had strategically placed urinals throughout the house--two in the bedroom and one in the laundry room. He could be sitting watching TV and all of a sudden say, "Jo, I can't make it!" So I'd run to the nearest urinal, help him pull down his lounging pants and Depends and hope to catch the flow, which usually had already started. Some- times you had a bit to clean up, and sometimes you had to change out the whole works--the disposable underwear and the lounging pants. I came to appreciate his disposable un- derwear and the brilliant person who created them. A close friend asked me, "Hey Jo, did it bother you to see your dad and help him go to the bathroom?" I thought about it and said, "After the first time it doesn't bother you anymore."

I had a job to do and I didn't have time to think about the
male anatomy. I'm sure a lot of older men are very modest,
but my daddy has always humbled himself and was very
thankful for the help.

I learned that my daddy had a set schedule of eating and
an extreme routine of meals. He had a huge breakfast, huge
lunch and a light dinner. Being a diabetic, Daddy would
try to control his blood sugar with diet so the evening meal
was mostly a small amount of chicken or tuna salad. Let me
see if I can convey this correctly; you NEVER have the same
thing two days in a row. Breakfast, for example, started
with cereal (four kinds are in the rotation) and half a banana.
While he ate that I would prepare eggs, a meat, toast or
biscuits, and juice. Each day was a different way to cook the
eggs (three ways on rotation), a different meat (four types on
rotation), a different bread (two on rotation), a different jelly
(four on rotation) and a different juice (four on rotation).
Lunch was a meat, a salad or slaw, two vegetables and light
dessert. There were lots of items on this rotation. Needless
to say, my daddy LOVES to eat and demands variety. And
if you tried to serve a sandwich at lunch, which for him is in
the evening meal category, you would get corrected. In the
four months to come, I would cook more than I have in 27
years of marriage! And one of my least favorite things to do
is—yes, COOKING!

Daddy taught me his daily schedule which was so exact

that it would drive most people crazy. He explained the
timing of his newspaper, "The Price is Right", his shower,
lunch, switching locations to relax in the back bedroom
after lunch, which lights you turn on and off throughout the
day, dinner, putting on pajamas, turning on the nightlight
in the bathroom, take his hearing aid out and going to bed
at exactly 9:00pm...with MANY more details in between. I
wasn't sure if this was just a man thing or if 83 years olds
find comfort in routine. And when things are off one beat
worry can set in.

The toughest part to learn was taking care of Daddy at
night. I slept in the front bedroom across from Daddy's
room. This room had twin beds with mattresses that were
over 50 years old! The better of the two had a slope in the
center. Camping on the ground might have been more
comfortable, but I had to remind myself to be thankful and
"it's not about me." For the first month Daddy would have
to get up three times a night to go to the bathroom. I figured
a lot of this was out of fear and worrying about Mama. I can
remember being in a deep sleep and hearing "Jo! I gotta go!"
I'd jump up from bed and go in his bedroom, grab the walker for balance and grab the urinal, all while trying to keep
him from falling. Some nights I'd think, "Lord, how can this
much pee come out of one man!" Some nights we'd have
to change his clothes and disposable underwear, and sometimes I could put him right back to bed. After emptying the

urinal I'd head back to bed. I'd lie back down and my heart
would be racing. Just having to wake up and be on cue
so quickly and then trying to go back to sleep was hard…
then there was the pressure of trying to sleep not knowing
when you'd be up again. It was as if I was back on a nursing
schedule with a baby--up and down, up and down, with no
uninterrupted sleep. Daddy was an early riser, so at 6:00am
I'd be up with him to begin another day--exhausted. How
did my mother do this for so many years? And how did she
do it with a good attitude?

• • • •

On June 8th, my friend Debbie called from Murfreesboro
and said, "What do you need?" Debbie knew exactly what
it was like to be a caregiver. She had taken care of both her
parents until they passed, so she knew the physical and
emotional challenges of this assignment. As my mind raced
the only thing I knew I wanted and needed was a journal.
What was odd about this request is: I'm not a "journaler."
In the past several years of teaching women's Bible studies,
I wrote or typed a lot, but that was mostly in research style.
I love to research a Biblical subject, look up words in the
dictionary and even dig further into the Hebrew or Greek
meanings of words. I especially love to mark in my Bible!
Pens, highlighters and pencils are like colorful graffiti in my
Bible. Words to the sides of Scripture, thoughts in the mar-

gins and famous quotes cover it. I have even put the blank
places in the maps section to good use. But as far as sitting
and putting my feelings or thoughts on paper, well, that
wasn't a common practice. I admit the first of every year
I'd hear from other respected believers how much journaling helped them sort out feelings or process emotions. Or
I'd hear how they loved to look back at their journal and see
how God had answered prayers. So with good intentions I'd
buy a very attractive journal and attempt to write in it every
day, which, sad to say, would only last two to three days.

But this particular day all I wanted was a journal. Debbie asked, "Any particular kind?"

"No, you pick it out for me, and I know it will be perfect."

Within hours Debbie had bought a few items for me,
driven to Shelbyville and was knocking on the back door.
What a friend! She had a history of being the best gift giver
and this day was no exception. She had a Christian tote
bag for my short trips back and forth, some delicious food,
and the most beautiful red leather journal. Embossed in the
leather were trailing flowers and in the upper right hand
corner was the word FAITH. I knew instantly this precious
gift would be my companion, my new friend, and my outlet
for emotions.

After a short visit Debbie and I hugged goodbye, and I
thanked her for being such a great friend. She also told me,

"Anytime you have questions during this process, please call me...I've been through it all." I wasn't sure what that meant, but in the days ahead those words would become crystal clear.

That evening I decided it was time to begin. It seemed different than all the other countless journaling attempts. I wasn't approaching this lovely book as an opportunity to start a new habit. I was grabbing it as a means of need for my soul because the emotions were building up quickly in me, and they had to go somewhere. So I wrote my first entry:

Journal Entry | June 8th

Lord, I desire to be transformed. I'm sorry I raised my voice with Daddy. I was trying to win a battle and make a point which was unnecessary. I'm thankful for my parents. They are wonderful. I know in my heart I need to be a servant to them, with a willing and thankful heart. I'm so sorry. Help me. Teach me your ways as I do this job.

As you can gather from the entry, I had argued with Daddy. I was trying to be logical and he was being emotional. It brought back memories of growing up when we didn't see eye to eye. But regardless of age--8, 18 or 48--respect for your parents is always required.

• • • •

It was hard knowing that my mother was having surgery and I was not there sitting in the waiting room. But Aunt Mary and Cousin Dawn were faithful to give me the play by play. The doctor decided to only do surgery on the left leg. The right leg was the worst break, and there was lots of swelling which could cause infection if surgery was attempted. It was also dislocated, which took three tries of pulling before they got it back into place. So the doctor "stabilized" the right leg, and in three weeks she would have to go back and have the second surgery. After staying a few days at Vanderbilt it was decided she would be moved back to Shelbyville to Glen Oaks Rehabilitation and Nursing Home. This meant I could take Daddy for visits and she could rehab there as well. I thought to myself, "This is a good plan, and after all, with God's healing and my mother's effort she'll be home soon…then I can enjoy my summer!" At the time this seemed like a practical and also faith-filled statement. I didn't have a clue that it was really a statement of selfishness.

• • • •

After just a couple of days living with Daddy I realized, "Wait! I better check their bills!" This was another scary thing to jump into, but there was a comfort mixed in this

too--my mother is super organized! So I went into another
bedroom where she keeps her files, and it didn't take long
to figure it out. I had her checkbook, so I could look at the
previous months to see the pattern of bills. Now you have
to realize that this was not something I could ask my daddy
about if I had a question. Ever since I was a little girl there
were two distinct roles my parents had which worked well
for them. As I mentioned, my daddy did all the grocery
shopping. My mother handled all of the finances. My daddy didn't want to discuss money, savings, CDs, insurance,
etc.… It made him nervous and confused, so my mother
took care of all of it. As I studied her folders and binders I
realized she was very "diversified." She had a little money
here and a little money there. I suddenly remembered meeting her at the bank years ago at her request to sign their
signature card on all their accounts. She also had me sign
a Power of Attorney with their lawyer. At the time I didn't
think one thing about it. But now I was so thankful for my
mother's planning ahead and being so smart. I checked with
the banks to make sure I had signed the checks correctly.
With the POA I was able to add my name to their credit
card. I never thought I'd be praising God for my mother's
financial wisdom.

I also realized that I could not live with Daddy 24/7
because I would have to see my family and tend to my own
finances and personal matters. Within the first 48 hours of

the accident my cousin Dawn's sister, Tammie, called me
and offered to go over Mama and Daddy's long-term healthcare. She came over and we sat down at the kitchen table.
She looked over their policy and showed me the forms to fill
out and how to get the ball rolling on filing claims. She gave
me a crash course on Long Term Healthcare 101! Her visit
not only helped sort out questions and answers but brought
peace and hope. Dawn was helping Mama, and Tammie
was helping me. I will always be grateful to them. Their
timing was perfect. God truly sent them to me and I was so
thankful!

I realized with their insurance policy I could get caregivers to come help Daddy, allowing me some time to go home.
Evelyn, another family member, worked for a caregiver's
staffing company, so she came to my rescue and sat down
with me to talk about setting up caregivers to help. Just her
voice of encouragement calmed me down. Unfortunately,
with their insurance came a 90-day payout, which meant for
the first 90 days my parents would have to pay out of pocket
for any caregivers I used for Daddy. I knew this would be
expensive; so I met with their financial advisor, and she
helped me budget an amount to spend over the next three
months so it wouldn't cause a financial burden on my parents. We decided I could have three eight-hour days a week.
Now also realize that driving time to and from Murfreesboro
would cut out two hours per each eight-hour day. So basi-

cally, I was left with 18-hours per week to see Jeff and Mary Lee, pay my bills, run my errands and do whatever I needed to do. How would all of this work? What times and what days should I be gone? Will Daddy adapt to this?

When I read my devotional for June 10th I knew God was speaking to me by saying,

> *"Rest in Me, My Child. Give your mind a break from planning and trying to anticipate what will happen. Pray continually, asking my Spirit to take charge of the details of this day."*

Journal Entry | June 10th

Lord, keep me from any over-planning or thinking ahead when only YOU see the big picture. Help me Holy Spirit to stay connected to You. I really want to GET this; to be disciplined to stay connected and to talk to You. Help me! Thank you for helping my emotions today.

• • • •

Small towns tend to produce special characters and special people. Shelbyville was such a place and a wonderful place to grow up. It's a small town full of people with

big hearts. The church I grew up in was full of the most
generous, caring people…not to mention full of humor. My
hometown church was like the *Cheers* song, "Sometimes
you want to go where everybody knows your name." I
remember when I was growing up we sat on the same pew
on the same side of the sanctuary every Sunday. With the
same faces, same families and hearts full of love my church
was the epitome of hospitality. There were so many friends
of my parents that even now when I see them at age 48 I
feel like I'm 10 again. They always took the time to talk to
me, encourage me and love me at every age I reached till I
moved and married. So when word got out about Mama's
accident (word travels fast in a small town too) guess how
Daddy and I got blessed? Yep, FOOD! When each person
would come over to drop off food I would look at their
sweet faces and think, "You're older, but really you haven't
changed a bit." And they would just pour out that familiar,
genuine love I will always treasure. Seeing these familiar
faces flooded me with wonderful memories and reminded
me that God has blessed my family with a very special Body
of Christ in Shelbyville, Tennessee.

Along with the food came offers to sit with Daddy if I
needed to go run an errand or two. Until I could get my
plan together on caregivers I decided to take several precious neighbors and friends up on their offers. My first
break would be meeting Mama at the nursing home when

the ambulance transported her from Nashville. I knew
when I got to the nursing home I'd be filling out a lot of pa-
perwork and answering lots of questions; but, frankly, I just
wanted to see my mama.

I called Lavon and he graciously came over to sit with
Daddy so I could leave. Daddy didn't hesitate having the
company because he wanted me to check on Mama. It was
only a ten minute drive to the nursing home, and as soon
as I pulled in the parking lot, I saw the ambulance backing
in where they drop off incoming patients. As they rolled
Mama into the building I was shocked when I saw her legs.
The left was in a full black brace and the right was positioned in the most unusual contraption I'd ever seen. It was
this long "V"-shaped metal rod that was actually bolted into
her bones. The top of the "V" attached to the sides of her
thigh, and the point attached to the bone at the bottom of her
shin. In addition to keeping the leg stable it looked like she
could pick up cellular signals! Not only was I shocked, but I
was thinking that maybe she would not be coming home as
soon as I had hoped. This looked serious and ugly.

When Mama saw me she began crying, "Oh Honey, I'm
so sorry. I can't believe I've done this." Her face was so full
of regret, guilt and sorrow. I knew she was on heavy pain
medicine for her legs, but nothing was easing the pain of her
broken heart. For the last three years my mother had always
ended our phone conversations with, "Now don't you worry

about me and your daddy…we're doing just fine." I know
God tells us "Do Not Worry," but frankly, I couldn't figure
out any other emotion that applied.

As they rolled Mama into her room the ambulance guys
very, very, very carefully lifted her from the gurney to the
bed. It was so painful for Mama. I'm thinking, "How on
earth can she get comfortable with that thing sticking out of
her leg?" Several nurses stood around her bed with puzzled
looks on their faces. It's not every day a patient comes in
the nursing home with this thing sticking out of his or her
leg. It was incredibly awkward and clumsy to handle. They
propped both legs up on pillows and tried to position her as
comfortably as they could. The real trick was figuring out
how to assist Mama and not move that alien leg.

After we hugged and kissed a bunch and after she
apologized some more we talked about how Daddy was
doing, and I updated her on what I was doing financially. I
could tell she was a little loopy from the pain medicine, so
going over too many details would be a waste of time. As
we talked she stopped and said, "I've got to go to the bathroom." OK, I've got to see this. How are they going to do
this? I called for the nurse out in the hall and immediately
a nurse rushed in. She and Mama discussed the best way to
roll to her left side and stick a bedpan underneath her. Poor
ole Mama was having to hold it for a few minutes while the
nurse positioned the bedpan. Finally, she gave Mama the

green light to go. As the nurse stood on one side of the bed
with me on the other we waited and Mama...well...went.
Now as I share this next statement, please keep in mind that
Mama was on some serious pain medicine. With relief on
Mama's face she said, "Whew...that's so much better. I tell
you what...when I was at Vanderbilt and they took out that
catheter and I could just go freely...well, it was better than
any orgasm!"

What did she just say?! Did my 73-year-old mother just
say the "O" word? The nurse died laughing saying, "Lawd,
Ms. Gunter, I just knew you were going to say that!" WHAT?
EW! Well, I didn't know she was going to say that! I never
in a million years would have dreamed she would have
said that! Maybe in a couple of months I would remind her
of this moment. Or maybe I would just dismiss it from my
brain for the time being.

Leaving Mama was really hard but I knew I had to get
back to Daddy. He would be very anxious to hear how she
was doing and would want all the details. I told her I'd
bring Daddy for a visit the next day. She wanted to see him,
but she was also dreading it too. Before I left she wanted to
explain to me what had happened the day of her accident. I
patiently listened. She had just helped Daddy to their bedroom for his afternoon television/nap time. It was a beautiful day, and she thought it would be a perfect time for her to
sit on the back patio and just relax. But there was this tree

limb that was hanging over the patio. She had discussed
cutting it down with Daddy several times, but he didn't
like the idea of her doing it. Plus, he'd warned her not to do
anything stupid like climb a ladder and saw it down. She
said she thought, "He's settled in the bedroom, so I'll just get
that saw and take care of that limb…I'm tired of looking at
it." Then she thought, "Nah, I better not. I need to relax and
enjoy this beautiful day. I'll just call someone to come do it."
Then she thought, "Well, it's not a big deal. I can get the ex-
tension ladder and cut it right off." Back and forth she went
in her thoughts. She told me the mean ole devil tempted her
and the good Lord was trying to talk her out of it. Bless her
heart.

She described how she used the electric handheld saw
and how she turned and twisted, but the limb was being
stubborn. As she leaned to make another attempt the limb
gave way, and the weight of the saw pulled her from the ladder. As she started to fall she said she had a split second to
think, "Do I fall sideways? No, I could injure my shoulder.
Should I fall backwards? No, I could hit my head on the
patio concrete. I should just jump." So she threw the saw
away from her and jumped. But at 73 years old the mistake
was landing flat-footed on the hard ground. She forgot
about the osteoporosis in her knees. The shin bones shoved
into the knees and everything shattered. As I drove home I
thought about the accident and decided maybe I wouldn't

share it all with Daddy. I'd just hit the high points. I didn't want Daddy's blood pressure to go up since he was worrying enough already. I decided to talk about the positive points. It was a ten minute drive back home so I decided I'd better start thinking of some.

• • • •

After I thanked Lavon for sitting with Daddy and he headed home, Daddy was itching to get a report on Mama. "Well, she's good and bad. I think emotionally she's strong and knows there's a lot of work to do to get better. She's also feeling very guilty about the whole thing. When I take you to see her tomorrow, you're going to be surprised how her legs look. But the first surgery went well, and in a few weeks the doctor will do the second surgery." OK, how was that? It was direct...not a lot of details. In my heart I prayed, "Lord, please settle his emotions and help him be positive."

"Well Jo, I've been thinking. This is a terrible situation. And I could easily harp on Mama about how stupid it was to try and cut off the limb. But I'm not going to. What's done is done. I'm not going to mention it again or dwell on the 'what ifs.' We'll go see her tomorrow and just take things a day at a time."

If I was texting I'd say "OMG!" Where did that come from? Lord, thank you! Now that's the right attitude I was looking for! Don't know how long it will last, but for the time being, I'll take it and rejoice.

• • • •

That night, after putting Daddy to bed and removing his hearing aid, I decided to just sit quietly with the Lord and pray. My daddy is totally deaf in his left ear, and once his hearing aid is out from the right ear he's completely deaf. I know this is bad to say, but this was a blessing because no matter what was going on outside his bedroom--television, talking, music…hail, sleet or storms--my daddy was undisturbed until he had to pee, of course. Then I was disturbed.

As I thought about the past week, I realized I was exhausted and running on fumes. I was so tired emotionally. It's interesting--when you experience something traumatic that you've never experienced before you're extra tired. I guess you're spending so much time thinking about it, figuring out what to do and just flying by the seat of your pants, your energy is just zapped. The greatest enemy during this kind of experience is fear. You've got your own personal fears about your capabilities. Then Satan jumps into your brain with both feet and is constantly saying, "What are you going to do?" "How are you going to do it?" "How long is this going to take?" THEN he also challenges your spiritual side with, "Some Christian you are…you don't even want to serve your daddy!" "Can you believe God would do this and He didn't even prepare you?" "Aren't you angry with your mother for putting you in this situation?" THEN he switches sides and tries to get you into self-pity, "Bless your heart, you don't deserve this." "You shouldn't be expected to do all this." "Well, looks like this is where you'll be spending your summer." WHEW! If there was a switch to turn your brain off I would have done it. So many fears, so many unknowns...Lord, help me!

Jesus Calling | June 11th

"Trust Me and don't be afraid, for I am your Strength and Song. Do not let fear dissipate your energy. Instead, invest your energy in trusting Me and singing My Song. The battle for control of your mind is fierce, and years of worry have made you vulnerable to the enemy. Therefore, you need to be vigilant in guarding your thoughts. Your constant need for Me creates an intimacy that is well worth all the effort."

Journal Entry | June 11th

Lord, you are my strength and my song. Pick out a song, Lord, and bring it up today. Control my mind today, Holy Spirit. I need your insight, wisdom and intelligence. Help me watch out for fear. Thanks for letting me know it zaps my energy. Help me remember that my constant need for You develops intimacy with You.

No songs came to mind yet. So I trusted that when it was time, He would bring me a song.

CHAPTER THREE

Branching Out
and Being Stretched

O ne week had passed since the accident happened, and I was so excited about going back to the nursing home to see Mama and to also reunite her with Daddy. Up until this point I had not taken Daddy anywhere. He walks with a walker in the house, and I knew he had a transport wheelchair, but I'd never used it with him. First things first, after breakfast I asked him what he wanted to wear.

For years around the house, Daddy has always been in lounging pants and t-shirts. In my daddy's prime he always liked to dress very nice. When I was growing up, on

Sunday mornings my daddy would put on his suit and tie
then head to my brother's room to find Jed's wooden baseball bat. Then he'd walk through the house saying the same
thing every Sunday, as well as anytime he had to wear a suit,
"Well, I better take the ole bat to knock off all the women."
My mother would just shake her head as it to say it was the
most ridiculous thing she'd heard. Jed and I would laugh
every single time. In fact, when my daddy was a senior in
high school he was voted "Best Dressed."

Aunt Mary has always bought "Brother" really nice,
high quality shirts, so I thought I'd grab a couple and let him
choose. I knew Daddy wanted to look extra nice for Mama,
so the outfit had to be just right. He decided he would wear
a pair of khaki dress pants and a short-sleeve dress shirt
with a brown belt and brown shoes. But before he changed
into his dress clothes, he made his way on his walker to his
bathroom to freshen up. As long as Daddy could hold on
to the sink and steady himself he could do a lot on his own.
Sometimes he'd have to sit down and rest his legs a bit if he
stood longer than ten minutes, but he didn't mind because
he wanted to look and smell good. It's funny how older people want to describe what all they do to get ready...or maybe
it was just my daddy.

"Now Jo, I like to wash around my neck if I'm putting on a clean shirt. And this stuff I put on my face makes
my whiskers stand up. And I powder up so I'll be fresher.

Then, in a minute I'll finish shaving." I've never thought about describing the details of getting ready to anyone. I just do it. We'll see what happens when I'm 83!

He also started a routine with me that would be a daily ritual. After he would shave he would ask me to open the back door and blow out the razor shavings. Every time--every single time for the next four months-- he would say two things: "Jo, blow out my razor...Joe Frazier" and "Jo, please don't fall down the steps. If you fall and bust your head wide open, then I'll be in a mess."

This is just one of many routines we followed. Remember, my daddy is a routine guy with food, showering steps, daily schedule and with funny lines. Sometimes he'd just say, "Jo, get me my razor...Jo, what do YOU say?" And then my line was, "Joe Frazier." And every time he would laugh. And every time he'd tell me not to fall out the back door I'd reassure him I was OK and I'd be careful. Little did I know at this point, I'd have mornings to come when I wanted to hit something like Joe Frazier and just sling the razor out in the backyard. Lord, help me!

Two other questions Daddy would have for me when he finally finished in the bathroom were, "Jo, how does my hair look?" and "How do I smell?" Ever since I was a little girl my daddy has ALWAYS been particular about his hair. Heaven forbid it was windy outside. I can remember him checking with Mama, "Is my hair combed?" My daddy has never had complicated hair. It's snow white and short. And yes, it always looks exactly the same. So he'd say, "Jo, how does my hair look?" And he would prompt me that my line was, "Same as it always does." Then he'd laugh. As for the smelling part, there were about six colognes in the rotation, compliments again of Aunt Mary. And what was funny is they ALL smelled great. So he'd say, "Jo, how do I smell?" And I'd bend down just for the visual effect of him knowing I was actually (not really) smelling him and say, "Good."

So on went the dress shirt and pants, socks and shoes, and he finished with his belt. "Jo, how do I look?"

"Good."

"No really? Do I look OK?"

"Yes, Daddy, you look good." The tone of my voice over the next few months would change on this line too.

"Jo, go get my wallet so I can put it in my back pocket. And get me a fresh handkerchief. Since I don't have a butt, they help fill out the pants."

I didn't know what difference it would make since he would be sitting the whole time in the wheelchair, but I got them both. Then a simple truth hit me--a wallet will always be around, but in a few years the handkerchief will be extinct. Think about it. Who carries one anymore? Most twenty/thirty-something-year-old guys have never heard of a handkerchief. Just a side thought.

Before he would walk with his walker to the back

door, I'd ask him if he had to go to the bathroom. Since
Daddy wore disposable underwear there was about a three-
hour window of them staying dry. Most of the time he'd
say, "You know, I'd better try again." So on mornings we
would plan to see Mama I'd allow a couple of hours of getting ready time.

Going down my parents' carport steps was very
tricky. There are three steps, and they are very narrow-
-about half the size of my daddy's foot. After analyzing this,
I figured the best approach was for me to hold the door open
and then stand in front of him. Then I'd walk backwards
down the steps holding on to him. We would take it super
slow. I was so afraid he was going to fall. Later I would
ask my mama how did she ever do this without him falling.
She told me, "Well, we'd just take it slow. Now I'VE fallen
several times, but your daddy doesn't know it, so don't tell
him." I thought, "Now here lies a woman with two broken
legs, so would it really matter if he finds out she fell down
the carport steps a few times?"

Once I finally got Daddy loaded in the car I put the
wheelchair in the trunk and off we went. I knew Daddy
was excited and nervous at the same time. I was nervous
about him seeing the big "V"- rod sitting on top of her leg.
Oh well, whatever happens…happens. When we arrived at
Glen Oaks, I lifted the wheelchair out of the car and rolled it
around to Daddy's side. I'm embarrassed to say that I did

not know how to lock the wheels, but fortunately Daddy
told me what to do; and I immediately prayed, "Lord, please
don't let me ever forget this important step!" At this point
I also realized my parents' car had handicapped tags. No
disrespect to people who park in those spaces, but man, this
was a life-saver! Praise God for those spaces!

So there we went rolling down the hall to Mama's
room. We spoke to the nurses on duty and one of them
said, "Ms. Rhoda's been primping this morning because
she knew her husband was coming." We turned into the
room, and there lay my mother. She looked tired from the
stress and pain, but I immediately noticed she had put on
a little makeup and a little lipstick. Aw, that's so precious.
But not as precious as when Mama and Daddy saw each
other. When Mama saw Daddy she started to cry. I rolled
Daddy to her and locked his wheels. He quickly leaned
over, and she leaned over, and they gave each other several
kisses. She said, "Honey, I'm so sorry." He replied, "Now
don't worry, we'll get through this. You're tough as nails
and you'll be back." I'm not sure if this line sounded more
like a coach giving his player a pep talk, but she knew it was
a compliment. I felt like I was witnessing an intimate moment and needed to exit. It was just such a sweet moment
and it dawned on me, "My parents really love each other." I
mean, I knew they did, but now I was seeing them more as a
loving couple rather than just my parents. Even at the age of

48, seeing this made me actually feel all warm inside. They
talked and encouraged each other a lot which was nice.

Of course, as soon as Daddy focused on her legs
the "worry look" took over his face. She told him that she
had already started rehab on her left leg and that it was
hard. The right leg could NOT move until surgery, and we
hadn't heard when that would be. I noticed that my mother
could not be still. Since she was a woman who has always
been a doer, I'm sure just lying in bed was tough. She had
a room to herself, so she had an organized system of where
she wanted things to go. She was constantly rearranging
her legs, lifting them with her hands and propping them
on more pillows for elevation. I was beginning to wonder
if there would be a shortage of pillows in the nursing home
due to Mama's hoarding. She would sit up, and then lean
back, twist and pull, moving every second. I knew any
minute my daddy would pick up on it; and sure enough he
soon told her, "Mama, you're going to have to quit moving
so much…you're making everyone nervous!" Of course,
"everyone" really meant…him.

I was still hopeful that the swelling would go down
soon in her right leg and the surgery could happen maybe in
a week. Since phones were not in the nursing home rooms,
patients could have personal cell phones. So Mama had her
cell phone on at all times waiting on a call. But the doctor already knew when the surgery would happen because, well,

he is a doctor and is familiar with trauma breaks and how
they heal. The surgery would be in three weeks, meaning the
healing of her right leg would be three weeks behind that
of her left leg. Daddy and I left the nursing home, and the
drive home was a little quiet. I think Daddy just wanted me
to reassure him that things would be OK, but I was having
a hard time believing it myself. I had no doubt my mother
would give 110% with rehab, but the body has its own healing time frame. She could excel as a patient, but those legs
had to mend from the inside out. In the mean time, I had a
job to do. I had to keep going and take care of Daddy just as
Mama did. For 24 hours a day I was on call.

The days were the same, and you could actually
write out the routine hour by hour. When I tried to sit down
and relax I'd hear, "Jo?" It was reminiscent of what you see
in a movie when someone has almost reached the seat of the
couch, and he or she has to stop in mid-sitting position to
go see what was pulling them away. Sometimes he needed
help going to the bathroom; sometimes he wanted a piece of
chocolate; sometimes it was just to show me something on
television. After the first week I realized I was in Bill Mur-
ray's movie *Groundhog Day*. Every day the same…same
chores….same funny lines…same meals (with rotations
added of course)…same clothes…same everything. Even
though I loved my daddy and I knew this was exactly where
and what I was to be doing for a season, one thing was for

certain—I wanted to go home. I missed MY family.

• • • •

Journal Entry | June 14th

This morning I sat outside and cried to the Lord. Not out of sadness, pity or worry. Just a release. To just be with Him and to watch the beautiful redbird bathing in Mama's birdbath.

Sitting outside on Mama's patio was like heaven, especially on a beautiful summer day. Scanning over Mama's backyard, I took in the sight of every flower, tree, shrub and decoration. Wow! My mother knew how to landscape. It wasn't a perfect, manicured yard like you would expect from a professional landscaper, but it was a yard groomed with a true love for the outdoors and things that bloom. It felt comfortable and peaceful. I wished I had noticed it years earlier. I had thought my summer would be sitting by a pool with Mary Lee, but I decided to be grateful for the limited time alone that I was getting.

The birds really love Mama's yard because she has blessed them with a birdbath. I especially love seeing redbirds. They just seem to really minister to me. Years ago I was sitting on my back patio praying and needed the Lord

to confirm that He was listening to my prayers and that
He loved me. Suddenly a redbird flew up and landed on
the top of the patio chair in front of me. I tried so hard to
be still, but it shocked me and delighted me all at the same
time. He only stayed for a couple of seconds, but for me it
was a precious blessing from God, and it confirmed that He
did love me. Moments outside weren't an everyday routine, but when I would get the chance to sit outside I would
have to go back in the house every fifteen or twenty minutes to peek on Daddy. Possible breaks were always in the
afternoon because that's when he would relax in the back
bedroom in his recliner and watch a baseball game with an
occasional "catnap" too. I learned real quickly that if he saw
me I'd hear, "Jo! Let me ask you something." Or sometimes
he would just want to tell me a story. Although my daddy's
stories were very funny I had pretty much heard each one
thousands of times; and even though I usually didn't mind
hearing them again, I just needed a break from talking, listening and thinking.

One afternoon I branched out and decided I had
to exercise and get some fresh air. I just needed a good
walk around the block. I asked Daddy if he would mind if
I took about a thirty-minute walk; he didn't mind at all. I
made sure he did not have to go to the bathroom and even
told him, "Now Daddy, don't get up. Just stay put till I get
back." He said, "Oh, I'll be fine. You go ahead...and Jo, be

careful." So I suited up in t-shirt and shorts, and put on my
tennis shoes, and out the door I went. I can't tell you how
excited I was. It was like I was on an adventure. Throughout the walk I called my cousin Dawn. During this whole
situation with Mama's accident my cousins Dawn and
Tammie were also dealing with their parents. My Uncle
Haywood, mother's brother, was going downhill quickly in
his health, while my Aunt Betty had suffered for years with
Parkinson's disease, as well as other health issues. Because
of my aunt and uncle's long-term healthcare insurance they
had caregivers around the clock, but still my cousins had
their hands full with doctor visits, errands, bills and staying
the night with them frequently, not to mention the mental
weariness that I was already experiencing. These two had
helped me so much over the last week, but because I had
never experienced taking care of a parent, I had no clue what
they had been going through over the past year. I was so
humbled. Lord, please forgive me. Uncle Haywood was not
doing well at all, so as I walked I thought Dawn and I could
encourage each other over the phone. As we talked she
cried, so I just prayed for her out loud and asked God to be
merciful with Haywood. *"Lord, don't let him suffer and bring
peace to him and his body. Also refresh Dawn and Tammie and
help them rest in You."* Just her sharing with me her and Tammie's experiences strengthened me, letting me know I could
do this and that it wasn't as bad as it could be. If they could

do it then I could do it. I wanted to honor my daddy and be
the best servant and daughter I could be.

When I walked in the house and took off my shoes
I immediately headed to Daddy's room to check on him.
Before I even got to the hall I heard, "Jo, I fell." I sprinted to
the bedroom, and sure enough, there sat Daddy on the floor
in front of his chair. Urine was everywhere! He had to go
and decided he would be OK to stand on his own and go
all by himself. Logistically, I don't know how he was in the
position he was in on the floor. He should have fallen forward, which meant he would have hit his head on the corner
of the television stand. All that was hurt was a bump on his
hand. I could feel my heart racing as I asked over and over,
"Daddy, are you OK? Did you hit anywhere else? Did you
hit your head?" He assured me he was fine.

Finally, I began to calm down and thought, "Now
what do I do?" I told him not to move, and I ran to get a
towel to soak up the puddles on the floor. The next challenge was getting him back into the chair. Fortunately, he
had fallen AFTER he had pulled his pants up, so I concluded
that he had dropped the filled urinal while falling. My mind
was racing and I started praying in my heart, "Lord, You
obviously had big angels on standby while I walked. Now I
need them to help me get Daddy back in the chair."

I knew the rule, "Don't Lift With Your Back, Lift With
Your Legs." I have pretty strong arms and legs and physi-

cally I'm in good shape, so I should be able to do this. "Alright Daddy, when I lift under your arms you use the bed to push yourself up." He said, "OK," but he didn't have a clue what I meant. I understood what my mama had told me about how it was getting harder and harder for Daddy to logically think things through. It was like he had lost the vision of how to do simple steps. Or as my mother would say, "Your father has no imagination." Maybe this was part of the affects of dementia? After the first couple of tries it was like trying to lift a tree log! He was completely dead weight. Well, now what do I do? Do I go to plan B? Actually, what was Plan B? Should I call the police? Should I call a neighbor? But I didn't want anyone hurting their back. *"Lord, we have no Plan B, so You are going to have to help me."*

"Daddy, let's try it again. I need you to really use your upper body to push up on the bed and the chair." I gave it all I had and finally he was up in the chair. It wasn't a pretty sight, but we did it. I remembered stories my mother would tell about Daddy falling, so now I had experienced it firsthand. Again the same question would come to me, "How did my mother do it?" I thought about her standard line at the end of our phone conversation, "Now Honey, don't you worry about us...we are just fine." So this was "fine?" Wow, I was realizing more and more that Mama was such a positive person and so strong that she confessed this statement all the time. She could have eas-

ily complained, but she took life as a caregiver one day at a
time. The "respect-odometer" was going up and up for my
mother every single day I lived with Daddy.

• • • •

    After Daddy's outing to the nursing home it was
clear that we needed a wheelchair ramp at the house. I
could not risk Daddy falling down the steps, and with
Mama coming home one day soon, she would need it too.
I petitioned God and asked Him to show me what to do.
Mama and Daddy's money was tight, and after a few calls I
found out insurance would not pay for it. After a few days
of praying, David, an old friend of mine, came to mind. He
and I had been close friends since fourth grade, and we grew
up in church together. He was like family. I knew David
would know who to call and what to do. I called him and
found out he had heard about Mother's accident. As we
talked I couldn't help but get upset. I could tell my emotions
were so tender and it seemed like any conversation I would
have with anyone would result in tears. But what could
I do? When I asked David if he knew anyone who could
build a ramp, he immediately said, "Yes! In fact, he is here
at my house working on some projects. How about I bring
him over tomorrow and you show him what you need?" I
was shocked and so excited.

    "Now David, I'm working with a budget, so help

me get a good price." Are you kidding me? A "budget?" I didn't have a clue what a ramp cost, nor did I know how much I could spend of Mama and Daddy's money. I was truly stepping out on faith and trusting God and hoping God was telling David my imaginary "budget."

The next day David drove up with a local contractor. He was a soft-spoken man, who looked like he knew exactly what he was doing. I could tell he was the kind of guy who could not only build anything, but who paid attention to every detail. As we walked around the house and looked at the options, he suggested the best location should be to build the ramp going out the front door. We could have built out the back patio door, but I knew it would take more lumber, and I just could not mess up Mama's backyard and the heavenly view. Summer after summer my mother would work in that yard, planting flowers and moving dirt. As I sat outside on the patio and found peace watching the redbird in the birdbath and beholding the beauty of Mama's hard work, I just couldn't throw a big ramp there. When Mama comes home, she will need that familiar haven again. So outside the front door it would go. In two days the contractor would start. I didn't know what it would look like and I still didn't know the cost. Daddy would ask me, "Jo, what's this going to cost us?" I would tell him, "I'm not sure, but David knows our budget." This line helped because I knew the last thing Daddy wanted to talk about was money details. He was trusting I knew what I was doing, and I was trusting God that David knew what they were doing.

At this same time I decided to use a caregiver to watch Daddy while I went home. Evelyn took the time to find the right person, and he was perfect. E.B. was a mountain of a man with a heart of gold. He came over one day to meet Daddy. As we sat and shared, I knew he would be perfect. E.B. loved history, baseball and a good laugh, which were all of my daddy's top three favorites. I felt very good about this. I decided to leave the house at 1:00 pm and come back to Shelbyville in the evening. The morning of my first planned getaway I was very nervous. This was a big day, and E.B.'s first day to sit with Daddy. This was also the first day of the ramp being built. What was I thinking? Actually I decided not to think, but when it was time I would just drive off!

When I left the house Daddy seemed content and the contractor was hammering away. My adrenaline was pumping and my heart was racing. I was leaving my daddy with a stranger and I was entrusting a man to build a ramp that I didn't know the cost, nor what it was going to look like. All I knew was I was going home and in the midst of a nervous body, I had peace.

Walking in my house was so wonderful, yet I felt like I had been away for months. It smelled so good. You know how everybody has a natural scent? Well, I could smell the sweet aroma of my husband, Jeff, Mary Lee and even my 20-lb cat, Solomon. It smelled familiar and wonderful. I sat on my red sofa and just rested. I cried some. I walked around some. I was home. As precious as this moment was there was also a slight sadness that in a few hours I would have to head back to Shelbyville. But for now, I could be Jeff's wife, Mary Lee's mama, and enjoy the moment. That evening we ate with our best friends, Kelly and Cindy. Seeing them was equally as wonderful. They were so sweet to me, telling me we could go wherever I wanted to go. I felt like it was my birthday and all eyes were on me, which made me feel special. It was a reminder that God had blessed our lives with the greatest friends.

Journal Entry | June 15th

Thank you, Lord, for an evening out. Guide my time.
Direct me when and how often to get a caregiver.
Thank you for E.B.

Leaving Jeff was so hard. As I got in the car and started to drive to Shelbyville I couldn't help but cry. It was like living in two different worlds. I knew as I entered Shelbyville I was back on duty and needed to put my game face on again. I was curious how Daddy did with E.B., and I was even more curious how the ramp looked. *"Lord, please let it look good."*

As I pulled in the driveway about 9:00 pm, the car faced the house, and I took a deep breath and hit my high beams. The only scripture that perfectly fits what I saw was:

"Now all glory to God, who is able, through His mighty power at work within us, to accomplish infinitely more than we might ask or think."
Ephesians 3:20

I couldn't believe my eyes. It was the most beautiful thing I'd seen. It was perfect. So guess what I did? I cried. *"Lord, You have outdone Yourself. Thank you."* I couldn't wait to see it at daylight and to call David. When I walked in the house I could hear E.B. and Daddy in his bedroom talking. When I entered the room Daddy was smiling. The day and evening had gone well. As I walked E.B. to the door, he assured me they did just fine and that Daddy was very entertaining, as I knew he would be. Daddy had told lots of stories, which are always funny. E.B. was the ideal caregiver I needed for Daddy for the time being.

Although Daddy likes to go to bed at 9:00 pm sharp, he was full of questions and comments. He liked E.B. and said they enjoyed each other. He talked about how he could hear the hammering going on and how E.B. would go outside and check the progress. Since E.B. had a construction background he knew the contractor was doing an amazing

job and felt this was the Cadillac of ramps. I told Daddy
we would check it out the next morning. Daddy talked and
talked and I just let him. After a few minutes I could tell he
was winding down and was ready for bed. This had been
a big day, and tomorrow we would go again to see Mama.
As I tucked him in and started to remove his hearing aid
he said, "Jo, E.B. is a nice guy...but Jo, I missed you. But I
understand you have to see your family too. But I want you
to know I missed you."

I just smiled, bent down and kissed his forehead. "I
missed you too, Daddy. Goodnight, Daddy."

"Goodnight, Jo. I love you."

"I love you too, Daddy."

For years as a little girl he had kissed me goodnight,
tucked me into bed and said, "I love you, Jo." Now the roles
had switched. As I walked out of his bedroom, I told the
Lord, "Thank you for letting me now be the one to tuck him
in."

• • • •

The next day I couldn't wait to see the ramp! Even
after getting up three times with Daddy throughout the
night, I was wide awake and ready to see this beauty. After
breakfast I put Daddy in the wheelchair and rolled him to
the living room, and I opened the front door. Wow! Daddy
said, "Gol-lee, what a ramp!" He spoke the truth--now this

was a ramp. It still needed sanding and handrails, but its
unfinished form was awesome. After I settled Daddy in his
den chair with the morning paper, I called David.

"David, it's just beautiful. It's so amazing. It's better
than I ever dreamed. Now David, how much will I owe the
contractor?"

"Nothing. You don't owe a dime."

"What? David, you can't do that!!!"

"Well, yes I can. Look, I'm not doing this for you.
I'm doing this for Ms. Rhoda. I love your mama and I want
to do this. Listen Mary Jo, I have the resources to do this and
I want to...So how you like them apples?"

David has always had a way with words and with
"sayings."

"I don't know what to say."

"You don't have to say anything. It's my pleasure."

There was a slight silence as I couldn't talk choking
back tears. David knew there was not any more to say. He
knew, and I knew that this kind of gift could not be paid
back. As a Christian man, David knew the joy of giving.
He delighted in doing this and I just had to let him. What
a beautiful, loving seed David had just sown; and we both
knew that reaping from God far outweighed any payback I
could offer.

Later that day I knew what I could do for David. I
could pray blessings over him and his wife, Tanya, and

over their family and business. I could ask and believe God to bless him with a hundredfold return on his investment for my mother. So I texted him a prayer and asked God to continue to richly prosper them, so they could continue to be a blessing to others in need. The Lord actually helped me compose the perfect prayer with a perfect ending--"So how you like them apples? Amen."

CHAPTER FOUR

A Longer Journey

Over the next few weeks I had good days and bad days. There were days Daddy would be humorous and days he would just be on edge. Each day was the same routine, yet emotionally unique.

Jesus Calling | June 17th

"Don't take yourself or your circumstances so seriously. Relax and know that I am God with you. When you desire My will above all else, life becomes much less threatening. Stop trying to monitor My respon-

sibilities – things that are beyond your control. Find
freedom by accepting the boundaries of your domain."

Journal Entry | June 17th

But Lord, all of this IS serious. So is this Your will for
me? I don't mean to be a spoiled brat but is this my
path? I guess I am monitoring your responsibilities
instead of just letting go. You'll have to help me find
freedom in this. And the joy too.

Getting up with Daddy, night after night, was the
hardest part. One night he decided he wanted some chicken
noodle soup for supper. That was very easy to fix. Grab
the can out of the pantry, open the can, heat it up and serve.
Now this was my kind of cooking. Well, "easy to fix" backfired on me. Daddy was up that night at 11:30 pm, 2:15 am,
5:15 am and 6:30 am. He felt so badly that each time I had to
hold him steady. Each time he would say, "Jo, I'm so sorry.
I shouldn't have eaten soup." I'd say, "It's OK, Daddy." He
would just shake his head, like he was disgusted at himself.
At 6:30 am as we stood together while he was going in the
urinal he said, "Jo, I've decided I want soup for breakfast."
With his hearing aid out he couldn't even hear me laugh. I
was exhausted, but that was hilarious.

One night after I had helped Daddy at about 2:00am,
I decided I might as well go to the bathroom too. As I sat

there, I studied the toilet paper and thought, "Hmmm…is this one-ply or two-ply?" Then reality interrupted my thinking. Oh my gosh! Lord help me! I'm sitting on the commode in the middle of the night dissecting toilet paper. What is happening to me?!

Still another night, I heard him say, "Jo! I gotta go!" I was in such a deep sleep and in the middle of dreaming. I jumped up and rushed in the room and quickly realized my hand was asleep. Have you ever tried to hold a urinal with a numb hand? I prayed, "Lord, please don't let me drop this…please don't let me drop this." It was only by the grace of God that I was steady. Thank you Jesus!

Journal Entry | June 18th

I was up at 2:00 am, 4:30 am, then at 6:15 am. My goodness…where does all that pee come from? I'm so tired. But as I stood there at 6:15 I told the Lord, "How can I keep doing this?" He whispered, "Do it as unto me and I will reward." This morning a friend sent me a text with 2 Chronicles 15:7 that said, "But as for you, be strong and courageous, for your work will be rewarded." I truly love when God confirms with His Word.

• • • •

Day after day, Daddy and I would get more comfortable with each other, and I don't mean that was always in a positive way. Since Daddy was a habitual worrier he would sometimes vent those worries to me. I knew each day he worried about Mama and how long it would be until she would come home. He would go from feeling sorry for her to asking me why she had to climb a ladder. He would voice how much he missed her, and in the next breath he would say how hardheaded she was. Sometimes I would try to reason with him with logic and a positive point of view, but he would shoot down both of my tactics. Negative people WANT to be negative. If someone is dead set on feeling like they need to complain and worry out loud, it can be irritating to them if you try to stop them. I also realized that me complaining about a complainer was just more still complaining!

<u>Jesus Calling</u> | June 22nd

"You are tempted to indulge in just a little complaining about My treatment of you. Thanking Me for trials will feel awkward and contrived at first. But if you persist, your thankful words, prayer in faith, will eventually make a difference in your heart."

Journal Entry | June 22nd

Lord, Daddy frustrated me so much today. First, he worries that we will have too much food from people bringing it and that it will go bad. Then he worries that we'll run out of food and I'll have to go buy more, which will cost money. Getting 30 cents off on gas today was a blessing, but when I told him I only had to pay $2.83 to fill up, he said that he guessed he and Mama were headed to the poor house. This hurt my feelings and I wanted to cry. I'm trying so hard to stay positive. Lord, please help me to stay thankful. Thankful for where I'm at and thankful for what You're doing.

"I will offer to You the sacrifice of thanksgiving. And will call upon the name of the Lord"

Psalm 116:17

• • • •

Three weeks had passed. I couldn't decide if they had passed quickly or slowly. When you're doing the same thing every day it seems so slow, yet you look up and weeks have passed. Every other day Daddy and I continued to go to the nursing home to see Mama. I got to know the nurses who I dearly loved. And oh, how they loved on my mother. She was there for rehab only, and they were dealing with a woman who was sharp as a tack and a joy to be around. I had never been around nursing homes very much. I remember while I was in high school, Mama's daddy was in a nursing home. Every once in a while I would go with her to see my granddaddy, and I just remember it being so depressing. The smell was nauseating, and seeing the residents was so sad. Now that I was going regularly I really got to see what these gifted men and women go through taking care of patients every day. I know there are lots of horror stories in nursing homes, but Glen Oaks Nursing Home was wonderful. The nurses worked hard, and I looked forward to seeing them every visit. God bless them for what they do and what they have to endure. I got familiar with the patients on Mama's hall, so when I wheeled Daddy in we would speak to everybody.

On the day after the ramp was finished, Daddy and I went to see Mama to share about the new addition to the house. Of course, we had to give it a test drive. Wow, this ramp rocked! Daddy was so impressed. He was proud of it. He was humbled when I told him that it didn't cost him a dime, so he could not wait to tell Mama. We would visit her about the same time of day, so each time she would be waiting for us with excitement and a smile on her face. I had barely parked Daddy next to her bed before he started telling her about the new addition. My mother cried as Daddy shared how David wanted to bless them by taking care of the expenses of the ramp. I showed her pictures on my cell phone. She was in awe and so thankful, yet I could still see the guilt on her face that said, "My accident costs others money!" She was still battling on the inside to forgive herself.

On days when Daddy and I didn't go to the nursing home Mama and I would talk on the phone...no, actually I talked to her every day. We both were using *Jesus Calling* by Sarah Young as our devotional, so we would encourage each other with it. If I was down, she would encourage me...if she was down, I would encourage her. Living at the nursing home wasn't easy, yet the Lord would always encourage Mama with surprises. One night she said she was really down on herself and depressed. It was late at night and usually this 80-year-old man down the hall starts yelling, "ICE WATER!!" The nurses would try to get it to him as soon as they could to quiet him. It was like an evening ritual. On this particular night however, he didn't yell....he sang... he sang at the top of his lungs "Jesus Loves Me." She said the nurses just let him sing. For Mama it was beautiful and encouraging. She said she and Jesus just had church right there in her room. I was humbled by how the Lord ministered to my mother that night.

• • • •

Mama had made great progress with her left leg in the two weeks after her surgery. The physical therapists were amazed by this 73-year-old's determination and stamina. She would wake up in the middle of the night and do leg lifts or upper body weights. She didn't ask herself how she felt; she just continued to do the rehab. I had been praying that her rehab would be over quickly and above normal, and so far that's what was happening. She found out that the doctor was ready to do surgery on the right leg, and boy was she excited. No more V-rod! I was nervous and excited too. So far I had no time frame on her recovery and when she could start standing again. Would she do rehab at Vanderbilt after this next surgery?

I made the decision that since I had missed the first surgery I would be there for the second one. I was looking forward to meeting the doctor myself, and I had my list of questions in my head. With help from a family friend and E.B., the entire day and evening were now covered. David and Tanya had invited us to the Boys and Girls Club Celebration Banquet in Shelbyville on the evening of the surgery. Kelly and Cindy would be attending as well, and I desperately needed an evening out, so my plan was to meet Jeff at the banquet for a nice dinner and fellowship after Mama was in recovery. As I drove to Nashville I was mentally ready to spend the day at Vanderbilt. Mama would go by way of ambulance to Vanderbilt and the surgery was scheduled for June 26th.

Journal Entry | June 25th

Mama on her way back to Vanderbilt. You've prepared the way, Lord! Literally. Thank You that You're in charge of her and this surgery. Let thanksgivings be on my lips!

I texted my sisters in Christ, who for the last several weeks had continued to encourage me and pray for Mama's healing. They would always point me to Jesus with their calls, visits and texts. Their prayers kept me strong and focused. What a gift from God.

Jesus Calling | June 26th

"Stay calmly conscious of Me today, no matter what. Remember that I go before you as well as with you into the day. Nothing takes Me by surprise."

I thought it was funny that this was the theme of my devotional on the day of the surgery. Years ago, me and my prayer partner and dear friend Trish would get together several times weekly and just pray for people. When faced with

a situation of difficulty Trish would say, "Well one thing's
for sure, this didn't catch God off guard." I had used Trish's
line so many times when ministering to someone who was
suddenly dealing with a surprise life blow. I could hear myself say, "It's going to be OK; this didn't catch God off guard.
He has a plan and He is mindful of the whole situation." It
is easy to have great faith when ministering to someone else.
Now I would have to walk this out.

Mama was so glad that I was with her in the holding room at Vanderbilt. As they prepped her for surgery
and asked a million questions we talked about a little bit of
everything. She didn't seem nervous but more anxious to
get on with it. Then she saw her doctor outside the door. I
rushed to the hallway so I could meet him and ask my questions. Either I'm getting old or doctors are getting younger.
This young doctor was (I'm thinking) early thirties with
black hair and big brown eyes and quite handsome with a
wonderful personality. The first thing he shared with me
was in regards to the first surgery on her left leg. He said
she had about nine screws and one plate. He informed me
the right leg would require two plates, and as he put it, "a
bunch of screws" since the break was so bad. I finally asked
directly, "When will she walk again?" He plainly said, "Left
leg--she can put weight on it September 7th; right leg--not
until September 28th. She should be slowly walking by November, maybe end of October. She'll stay at Glen Oaks and

do rehab for three months."

I know my face looked like I was in shock. Is this what the word "devastation" feels like? It felt like someone had hit me with cold water. Did I hear him correctly? She couldn't even stand for three more months? She wouldn't be walking around till maybe November? My mind was racing. I wanted to burst into tears. I tried so hard to suck it up, but I couldn't. The doctor knew I was about to lose it. To be honest, at this point his lips were moving, but I don't remember one more word he said.

I'm not one who can hide my emotions very well, so attempting to put on a positive face with my mother was impossible. When she saw my face she immediately asked, "What'd he say?"

"Well Mama, you'll be at Glen Oaks for three months. You can't put any weight on your legs till September."

"You've got to be kidding? Oh honey...I can't believe this." She was about to go down the "I'm so sorry" road again and I stopped her.

"Now Mama, we can't keep doing this. I'm not mad at you; in fact, I'm so proud of you. But if it will make you feel better I forgive you. Now Mama, your line is, "I receive your forgiveness."

She looked at me with tears in her eyes and said, "I receive your forgiveness."

"Great! Now I don't want you to apologize anymore.

We are moving forward. We're taking a day at a time and it's going to be OK."

Leaving Mama so they could begin surgery was hard. I hated to give her all the facts right before they wheeled her in, but my mother has never liked having things sugar-coated or left in the dark. She likes to know the facts and now she had them.

I knew surgery would take several hours and Mama knew I would not be there when she woke up. She was so excited that Jeff and I were having an evening out of the house. My Aunt Mary was in the waiting room when I left the holding room. I filled her in, and she said she would stay as long as she could. One of my dearest friends Lisa came to Vanderbilt while I waited which blessed me so much. She has always made me laugh ever since we were in high school, and at this moment I needed to feel lighter. By the time I left Nashville Lisa had me smiling, and she paid for my valet parking because I had no money. A true friend.

The drive back to Shelbyville was long and tiring, perhaps because I was emotionally numb. I kept thinking about what Mama's doctor had said about her not even standing up until September and then not walking again until maybe November. And it was just the end of June!

As I drove to the location of the banquet, I just sat in my car a minute. My emotions were so raw. I just wanted to cry. I wanted to see my friends, but I had no appetite, and

I knew the first question people would ask was, "So how's your mother?" What do I say? "Oh, she's great! She has to lie in a bed for three months and can't walk till Thanksgiving." I consider myself a fairly positive person, but how do you spin this one? And I didn't want to be pitiful. I had two good legs! "Come on, Mary Jo," I told myself, "You can do this!"

Kelly and Cindy have known me so long that I knew they could read my face and know what I was feeling. And Cindy, being one of my best friends, knew that if she asked questions I would cry, so she didn't want to do that. I'm thankful we did not sit with them because we are so close that it would have been harder to keep it together. Seeing David and Tanya was a blessing. I shared with David what the doctor had said and strained to hold back tears. Words were getting caught in my throat, and my thoughts were foggy. I can't remember David's exact words, but he spoke words of faith and reminded me that my mama was tough. He was right.

Throughout the banquet I would just look at Jeff. He is so handsome. I was proud to be his wife. I never heard a word the speaker said. It's like I wasn't even there. All I wanted to do was crawl up in Jeff's arms and go to sleep. I needed him to tell me it was going to be OK. I needed him to hold me as tight as possible. I needed him to hum to himself, so I could lay my head next to his chest and hear it so it would drown my own thoughts and fears. Sitting beside my husband in a room full of wonderful people, I had never felt so alone.

As soon as it was over I was ready to bolt to the door and leave. I told Jeff good-bye and got in my car to head home…wait, no, not home…to Daddy's. Lord, I know I grew up there, but my home is in Murfreesboro with Jeff and Mary Lee. My home is not at Daddy's. Why was this debate in my head frustrating me? As I was about to pull in the driveway, I thought, "No, I just need some time with You, Lord." So I drove around the block and down the hill to a church. I pulled around to the back of the church and put the car in park. My first thought was that 30 years ago this was a place teenagers came to go parking. And now here I am crying out to God for help. Thoughts went through my head so fast, "What do I do? Should Daddy stay with Mama at the nursing home? Am I to stay with him for the next three months?"

As hard as I could, I resisted the questions pounding in my head and just focused on God. I took some deep breaths and let Him rest a sweet peace on me. That brief moment behind the church with Jesus was what I needed to have the courage and strength to go back into Daddy's house. Through tears and exhaustion I chose to thank Him and praise His goodness.

<u>Jesus Calling</u> | June 27th

"You have journeyed up a steep, rugged path in recent days. The way ahead is shrouded in uncertainty. Look neither behind you nor before you. Instead, focus your attention on Me, your constant Companion. Trust that I will equip you fully for whatever awaits you on your journey.

Journal Entry | June 27th

Today is better. I cried a lot this morning but its been very cleansing. I know, Lord, You are more concerned with changing me than my circumstance. I do want Your will. I'll do what You want me to do. When people say, "You can't take care of your daddy that long," I honestly don't think that's Your heart. I'm counting on You God to help me honor my parents. I'm counting on You to be Mama's biggest cheerleader in the nursing home. I'm counting on you to arrange time for me to get away and be with Jeff and get some sleep. And I'm counting on you to work out all the finances.

"Let the morning bring me word of Your unfailing love, for I have put my trust in You. Show me the way I should go, for to You I lift up my soul."

Psalm 143:8

• • • •

After a couple of days, Vanderbilt shipped Mama
back to Glen Oaks. Even after trauma surgery, they do not
let you hang around the hospital and heal anymore. It was
my day to go home, so E.B. sat with Daddy. I decided on my
way to Murfreesboro that I would time it just right to meet
the ambulance bringing Mama back to the nursing home.
The nurses were so happy to see her. They welcomed her
with hugs and encouragement, and they were equally excited to see the V-rod gone! Mama was still very woozy from
pain medicine; so when I walked in her room her first words
were, "Oh honey, I've done a terrible thing." I could tell she
was under the influence, so I thought this could be entertaining. So I asked what she did that was so terrible.

"I told the Vanderbilt people that we had long-term-
health-care. Was I supposed to say that?" She sounded like
a little girl who thought she had said the wrong thing. I just
smiled; and in my assuring parenting voice I said, "It was
OK to tell them. In fact, you can shout it from the rooftops
if you want to. You can tell anybody you want. It's not a
secret."

But her face remained worried as she said, "I mentioned going back to Glen Oaks to the Vanderbilt people.
Do you think that's why they kicked me out early? Do you
think they were upset?" Again the face of a little girl who

thought she had hurt someone's feelings. I assured her that Vanderbilt wasn't mad at her and that she had come back at the right time. When I knew by her facial expression that she was relieved in her mind, I kissed her goodbye, so she could rest and I could go home.

I drove rather quickly to Murfreesboro because my bed was screaming my name. When I got home I walked to my bedroom, took off my clothes and crawled in my bed. It was the middle of the afternoon, but I wanted my bed. It smelled like Jeff. It was wonderful and my long nap was heavenly.

When I awoke, Cindy called and asked if we wanted to get together for dinner. Kelly and Cindy have a beautiful home, and my favorite part is their back covered patio. It is inviting and comfortable, and we've shared some wonderful times with them on this patio. So what did I want to do? I just wanted to order pizza and relax with them outside. Just the thought of being there choked me up. I guess it was familiar to me, and I needed familiar. I needed to just chill. Sitting on that patio was so peaceful and made me happy. I could share, cry, or not say a word, and it was safe to do that with these special friends. It was like I wanted to stop time and sit there for weeks.

When eight o'clock came I knew I had to leave. It was hard to leave friends and to leave Jeff. As I drove back to Shelbyville I realized I had a choice. I could drive in

silence and allow my mind to wander and worry, or I could
praise and worship God! I had an uplifting CD called "Col-
lage" by a Christian group called The Katinas. These guys
know how to worship. So I popped it in, cranked it up and
sang at the top of my lungs. It kept me awake, and focused
on God, and encouraged me. The Katinas soon became constant companions on my commutes. Even when I didn't feel
like praising God all I had to do was turn on that CD, and
the presence of the Lord filled my car. I remembered asking
God weeks ago to give me a song. Well, he gave me a whole
CD! Praising and worshipping God is a powerful thing. It
gets your mind off yourself and on God. I had to do it frequently.

When I got home Daddy had already gone to bed.
E.B. told me that he and Daddy had a good night. He said
they had cut up a lot and Daddy had told many stories
about me and my brother, Jed. He said that Daddy sure
was proud of us. This humbled me. Before I went to bed I
prayed, "Lord, I want to be thankful for where I am, the role
I'm in and that I have been blessed with a wonderful, loving daddy. Even if he's Negative Nelly at times, he is still
thoughtful and appreciative of me being here. Help me to
honor my daddy and to appreciate this time."

• • • •

Now that I had a healing time frame on Mama there

was no doubt I had to resign my job at the school. My new
job was caregiver to Daddy. I had great peace about this, but
knowing I would not get to see Christine every day would
be hard. She was the funniest human being I had ever met,
and we had grown so close. She was more than a co-worker;
she was my friend--a special friend--one I looked forward to
seeing every day. I knew my job was probably the best at
the school, maybe not in pay but in duties. I knew someone
was about to benefit and be blessed from me leaving. I was
sad, but I knew it was time. I also knew that when I told
Mama that I would be resigning she would feel guilty. But
only God could help her with this. Jeff was sad about me
leaving my job too, but he also knew it was the right thing to
do. We both knew that we had to trust God as our financial
source and provider. I reflected back to 1994 when the Lord
called me home from a career position to being a stay-at-
home mom for 14 years. I watched God provide then and
He was faithful. It was time to go down that road again. I
also remembered that at the first of the year Jeff and I felt led
to drop the school's health insurance policy and get on Jeff's
company's plan instead. I could see now this was a move
directed by God. I decided I would try to joyfully embrace
this task knowing that God would reward and bless us. And
I would praise Him for this privilege of blessing my parents
by serving them with my time and love. This was my heart
and my confession. I also knew that I may have to remind
myself of this wonderful viewpoint maybe every second of

the day.

Journal Entry | July 1st

Well, I resigned today. Feels peaceful, sad, and
strange. I know it's Your will, but I'm still sad. I'm
sorry I've complained. It was the best job You've ever
provided for me. You hand-picked it. Then You took
it away. Funny how that works. I feel a little lost. I
know my time will be spent here for a while, but I just
feel without purpose. Maybe it's because now I'm not
making an income. Well, guess I have to trust You.
Lord, I ask You to prosper Jeff and give him great favor
with clients. Encourage him Lord, and let him succeed
at the work of his hands. Bring him joy in his job as
well as prosperity. Strengthen me daily Lord because
You know I get weary.

CHAPTER FIVE

CHAPTER FIVE

Long Hot July

B y the first of July I had a routine in place. Maybe the sad part was--I had a routine in place. Every week, every day, every moment was the same. I had E.B. coming three days each week so I could go home for a few hours. Sometimes Jeff would come to Shelbyville to see me on a Saturday night with a pizza and a nice bottle of wine. Even though I'm a one glass girl, that glass and a few slices of pizza were delicious. The hardest day was coming back to Daddy's from home on Friday nights because I knew that the next time I would be back with Jeff and Mary Lee would be the following Tuesday. So weekends were tough.

As the heat of the summer was setting in it was too hot for me to sit outside for afternoon breaks. Like King David in Psalms 42 and 43, I continuously tried to encourage myself in the Lord. I would feel guilty for not wanting to be there and guilty for even having those thoughts. Then I remembered what my friend Debbie said in the beginning of this journey, "Anytime you have questions during this process please call me...I've been through it all." I thought back to the time she took care of both her parents. I can remember praying for her because I knew she was tired from caregiving, but I didn't truly understand until now, so I called her with my "feeling" questions.

"Debbie, did you ever feel guilty because you didn't want to be there?"

"Yes, all the time. Satan will make you feel like you're a sorry Christian for feeling that way. But it's OK; don't let him get in your head. You're going to have a lot of emotions during this time, mainly because you miss your own family and your life. Don't beat yourself up. Just take it a day at a time."

She also sent me a text message one day that I locked in my cell phone and referred to often.

> *"Praying for you today! I totally understand where you are. I pray the presence of the Lord overtakes you today, filling you with His peace and joy! I found*

making myself listen to praise music made it easier to offer a 'yet' praise which really does chase away the oppressive spirit that presses in when you're isolated in the midst of the situation(Psalm 42). The enemy never misses an opportunity; but greater is he who is in you to overcome!! It's only normal to miss your family and life and to grieve the time lost with them; but trust in God's faithfulness to pay back all and more that the locust have eaten and to watch over each of you thru it all!!! It truly may be the hardest thing you've ever walked through but God will prove Himself strong and in control in ways He never could have revealed to you otherwise! I came across this slip of paper in my Bible today that you gave me when I was in your shoes and it's Proverbs 3:5-6. May you walk with a heart full of trust along today's path, acknowledging Him in all you do! I love you, sister, and I'm lifting you up! :) :)"

Sisters in Christ are indescribable. They would call me, text me, bring me food; but above all, they would pray for me. What a difference prayer truly makes. God must have told them I needed it. My biggest female encouragers were my precious daughters. My oldest daughter, Ellen, lives with her husband, Joe, in Colorado Springs. Just one year ago at this same time I had been planning a wedding.

God blessed us with an amazing Christian son-in-law, who I like to call Prince Joseph. Ellen called me every day all summer. When I'd get in the car to drive home, I would call her on my cell phone and say, "I'm going home...wanna ride with me?" And she would always reply, "Let's go!" Some days our conversations would be full of laughter, and I would share with her the funny things her Papa would say. Other days she would have to endure my crying and slight complaining. She and Joe were faithful to pray for all of us every day. Mary Lee was my faithful texter. She would text me throughout the day, every day, "I miss you Mama, and I love you." She would text me pictures of she and my cat Solomon, because she knew pictures would help keep me connected. Mary Lee sometimes keeps things to herself; but Ellen shared that she called her crying one day, missing me at home. Ellen encouraged her to drive to Shelbyville and spend the night with me. She did, and it blessed me so much. Having her presence with me helped me feel like I was Mama again. Having her sleep in the bed beside me was such a great comfort.

Journal Entry | July 2nd

I'm down, or is this depression. I don't want to confess that. With the outside being so hot, there is not anything to do. Life here is centered around meals and urinals. I'm not complaining, Lord, it's just the way it

is.....Sorry had to stop writing because Daddy needed
a pee break. Ha. You know I trust you God, mainly
because You are good. Will You show Jeff Your good-
ness? I'll be OK, but I worry about him. Help him.

Journal Entry | July 4th

Well, it's the 4th – hot, dry and Jeff is going to the lake
with Kelly and Cindy. I'm OK with it. While I'm
here Lord, please work on me. Help my conversation
and my attitude. I want to be Holy as You are Holy.
I want to be free of judgment, sarcasm, complaining,
offense and fear. I want a heart and life full of love,
peace, gratefulness and compassion.

Daddy and I continued to make our every other day
visits to the nursing home to see Mama. I looked forward
to those days because it broke up the routine and seemed to
make the day go by faster. Wait...is that what I'm wanting,
for the days to go by faster? When I would think about September being the earliest Mama could put weight on her legs
it was overwhelming. September! I didn't know whether
it would be my new favorite month or a month I wanted to
be mad at! September 10th was when I would be finished
with the ninety-day payout on Daddy's claim. I could then
have more help and not have to pay any more money out of
pocket. But September?! Summer would be over by then

and Mary Lee will have started college. Should I do a mark-off calendar like Christine and I used to do with school days? Maybe Lord just help me enjoy each day and my parents' personalities. They are unique and quite funny. I'll even try to journal some of my favorites:

Journal Entry | July 4th

When Daddy and I left Glen Oaks, we were riding home and my mind was miles away. Then I realized that Daddy was talking and I was fake listening. So I decided to tune in to what he was saying. I couldn't believe what I was hearing. He was actually telling me about who he thought looked the best in their casket at the funeral home. You know, who looked more like themselves! It was like he was ranking them, and finally he decided on the top three. It was a fascinating observation.

Journal Entry | July 5th

Mama called me and said, "Now honey, please feel free to wear anything in my closet." Awe, that's so sweet. Of course I just don't think I'm going to be drawn to anything in my 73-year-old mother's closet. Not that Mama is frumpy or anything, but there's a slight difference in our tastes. I had to text this to Ellen and Mary Lee. They loved it! They think their granny is the coolest. They are right.

Journal Entry | July 5th

Old men fart a lot! And it's always when you are
walking behind them. And they think it's funny.
Lord, will my daddy ever grow up?

• • • •

My parents' pastor, Reverend Tom, called me as I
was leaving to go home on July 5th. He wanted to come
by and see Daddy for a few minutes. I didn't really know
Tom, but Mama and Daddy really liked him. When I told
Daddy he would be coming by the house, his response surprised me. Even though Daddy liked Tom, he didn't want
to be interrupted after he had settled in his bedroom for the
evening. He wanted to focus on the Atlanta Braves baseball
game, or on an old movie. I told E.B. to let Tom visit very
briefly. Since E.B. was such a big guy, I pictured in my mind
this bouncer--like at a bar--and when time was up, out the
door the Reverend would go! This was not a positive visual,
so I prayed all would go OK.

For some reason going home this time felt very
strange. I felt slightly out of place. I didn't like that feeling
at all. I didn't like the feeling of popping-in, then leaving

again. It made me sad. I wanted to stay joyful and to focus
on just being there, but all I could think about was everything I was missing by not living at home. I knew I had
to stay focused on being positive and thankful. I certainly
didn't want to be a "downer" every time I came home to
my family. I couldn't allow myself to think too much or
I would cry. I wanted to be strong. The hardest part was
realizing that this process would be for weeks...maybe
months. Every day and every week looked the same--same
routine, same meals, same pattern. Ironically, Daddy was
happy with the set-up. In fact, he had to have that routine,
but how long could I stand it. There were days I simply
craved different scenery. I would ask the Lord to help me
stay out of depression, and if I was close to that point to, to
please send someone to lift me up--to somehow send a word
of encouragement to me. One thing I would remind myself
of was how other caregivers experienced far worst circumstances and conditions than this. I had amazing parents and
a nice home to take care of Daddy. I had a wonderful family
and friends supporting me, and I had friends of my parents
encouraging me and bringing food. I had to remind myself
to look at this glass as being half-full.

    When I got back to Daddy's house E.B. told me that
Reverend Tom had brought communion. How awesome!
The next morning I asked Daddy about the evening. He
talked and talked about how much he appreciated Tom com-

ing over and how much he enjoyed taking communion. He said that Tom did such a wonderful job at explaining the cup and the bread, and how graciously he administered the elements. I was so thankful to God for pouring out His grace in such a special way, and especially for sending Tom.

On the same day, my mother was blessed by receiving some encouraging news. As you know, my mother had this accident because she wanted to cut down a tree limb. She is an exceptional woman--full of strength and determination. Therefore true to her character she was quickly becoming the "queen of rehab" at the nursing home. The supervising physical therapist realized how unique my mother was and decided to take over her case. My mother... she was a PT's dream! It's sort of like when a teacher finds a student who WANTS to learn. It is a rare case to find a 73-year-old who WANTS to do rehab, and WANTS to rehab more than is required. Mama told me this supervisor said that even though she was non-weight bearing that she could do so much more than just lay in the bed. She informed her that the next day Mama would be in a wheelchair working on more bending and circulation. My mother's voice was so excited. I knew she would be up at five o'clock in the morning ready to get started!

The PT pushed Mama by challenging her workout on her legs and arms. Mama told me one day she had worked really hard on getting to 15 repetitions in lifting her right leg.

When the PT came in the room for the session, Mama was so
excited to tell her the progress and that she had just finished
the fifteen leg lifts. The PT's response was, "well I didn't see
them...now show me." So Mama had to do them all over
again. Even though this lady was tough--my mama was
tougher and could rise to the occasion.

<u>Jesus Calling</u> | July 5th

*"Whenever you start to feel anxious, remind yourself
that your security rests in Me alone, and I am totally
trustworthy. You will never be in control of your life
circumstances, but you can relax and trust in My
control."*

Journal Entry | July 5th

*Hey-- just maybe-- the "scenery" is about to change!
One thing I knew was all of this was out of my con-
trol--the healing, the timing and the people God would
send. Nothing was in my control, but in my weary
state, this was a good thing and such a wonderful feeling.*

• • • •

    Living with a worrier can be tiring within itself. Daddy not only worried, but he has never been the handy man in the house. My mother fixed everything, and if she couldn't, she would make a call and get it done. One morning I was feeling very tired. I was also feeling cold symptoms were settling in on my body. I had gotten up with Daddy several times during the night; therefore I had no uninterrupted sleep. Needless to say, my mood was already on edge. My daddy noticed that the water in the sinks weren't draining as they should. He told me I needed to get some of that "drain stuff" and wanted to know how soon I could go get it. It seemed like every five minutes he would say, "Jo, now are you going to get the stuff for the drains?" Oh my gosh! How many times would I have to say, "Yes Daddy — I'll get it when I go to the store." He would immediately say, "Don't wait around and let it get worse." This happened to be a morning we were going to visit Mama, and then afterwards I would go to Murfreesboro. I knew there wasn't anything I could do until the next day, yet he just couldn't get it off his mind. In frustration I finally said, "Daddy, you get things in your head and over exaggerate everything!" Oh my goodness, he didn't like my response one bit. In fact, I think I hurt his feelings. He was quiet on the drive to nursing home.

The whole time we sat in Mama's room I couldn't
help but yawn and yawn. I was so sleepy. This was bad
timing because Mama was so excited about her new rehab
routine and here I am quiet from exhaustion and Daddy is
quiet from being upset with me. When we got back to the
house a friend of mine, Kendall, came by for a quick visit.
She had just gotten back from a year long mission trip where
she traveled all over the world in some of the most remote
places sharing the Gospel of Jesus Christ. She endured terrible weather conditions, bad health conditions, horrible eating conditions and unbearable sleeping conditions. I made
her share some of her worst times with me, so I could pull
myself out of my pity-party and hopefully receive a fresh
perspective. She prayed for me before she left, and I felt so
much better. God honored what I had asked of Him. He
sent me someone when I was getting down. He was faithful.

Even with my friend's encouragement, I still felt like
I couldn't get out of Daddy's house soon enough. I needed
to see Jeff, and I imagine Daddy was thinking he needed to
see E.B. instead of me for a few hours. When I got home I
just wanted to sit on my favorite red sofa and cry. Jeff was
so good to me. He sat quietly and allowed me to unload my
emotions. I truly felt like a mess.

Journal Entry | July 6th

All I want to do is cry. I can't seem to find content-
ment or joy. I'm wanting things to hurry up instead
of just living in the present. God, all I can think about
or process is the fact that I just want to go home.

Journal Entry | July 7th

It's a better day. I got a two hour nap and Daddy has
been so good today. He means well. Lord, I just need
more of You, to trust You with my time and to let You
do Your work in me. Lord, please help me be content
and understand that You have blessings for me daily--
right in the situation I'm in.

Journal Entry | July 8th

I just had to text Tammie and Dawn and say this,
"Due to the clogged sinks in the house, I've decided to
check MYSELF into Glen Oaks Nursing Home to stay
with Mama because it is a more positive and a less
worrisome atmosphere!"

OK, so maybe Daddy didn't over exaggerate about
the clogs. E.B. tried to fix the sinks and tubs, but it was just
getting worse. I finally surrendered and called the plumber,
Terry, a Christian man from Mama and Daddy's church. He
came to the house and worked and worked on the clogs.

The smell was pretty bad, which produced an obvious fret-
ting look on Daddy's face. He worried about the clogs, but
more so the cost to fix it. I didn't know what to do but pray.
The tension was getting heavy in the house and I thought to
myself, "It's just a clog…why do I feel so much pressure!"
I knew my prayer was to relieve me of stress from Daddy
more than to fix the clogs! I felt a little guilty about praying
so selfishly, but we both needed some peace. After a few
hours, the sinks were cleared! Praise God!

Terry shared with me about health issues he was
having, so I had the honor of laying hands on him to pray
for his healing. It felt good to set aside my concerns and
simply pray for the needs of someone else. It felt good to
just be a believer and pray. It took a day or two for the smell
to go away, but at least we were over this obstacle. I had
to reassure Daddy that even if Mama had not broken her
legs, the sinks would have still clogged, and she would have
called Terry. He finally calmed down.

• • • •

As God was teaching me so much while living
with Daddy, He was also teaching Mama. Day after day
of watching her and talking with her, I was so amazed by
her faith and courage. God was teaching her how to speak
words of faith and healing over her broken legs. She told me
that every day she would talk to her legs! It reminded me

of Ezekiel talking to the dry bones and them coming to life!
One day when I was visiting I had the honor of praying over
her legs and knees. It was a great moment...ME, MAMA
AND JESUS PRAYING TOGETHER!!

• • • •

As Uncle Haywood declined in his health, he lost his
ability to walk and went to Glen Oaks for rehab. He told his
family he wouldn't be going back home. Each day he was
there he grew worse and worse. Fluid built up in his body,
which caused his body to swell. He didn't talk very much,
but one of his quick conversations that Tammie shared with
me did make me laugh. He told her he wouldn't be going
home and Tammie told him, "Daddy, that is not your decision, but up to the Good Lord when it's time for you to go."
He replied, "Don't you think I've already talked to Him?"
I had no doubt he was ready and at peace about going to
heaven.

Isn't it amazing how God orchestrates things? Seriously, what are the odds that my mama and her brother
would be at the nursing home doing rehab at the same time?
I knew my mother would take advantage of this rare God-
appointment and be a blessing to him. My sweet mama
would wheel herself in the wheelchair down the hall to my
uncle's room about three times a day to visit and help him
with his meals. His fingers were so swollen, so she would

wash, lotion, and massage his hands, while talking to him. He liked it and in his few words would tell her how good it felt. I told her it was like Jesus washing the disciple's feet except she was washing hands. In the midst of terrible circumstances, God was using the opportunity to…well…be God. I didn't know how long Uncle Haywood would live, but one thing was for certain--the next few weeks to come was ordained by God.

Mama worked so hard every day with her rehab and getting stronger and stronger. She could dress herself in the bed, and she learned how to lift her body over into the wheelchair. She would roll down the hall to visit residents daily, in addition to seeing her brother. She would take occasional naps, but she never wasted time. She kept busy by knitting, talking on her cell phone to friends, and encouraging the nurses and patients. She brought Matthew 5:16 to life in the nursing home -*"Let your light shine before men, so they will see your good deeds and praise your Father in heaven."* She tried to stay positive and knew things could be a lot worse.

One of the things she was excited about was her next visit to Vanderbilt. She would have another x-ray on her legs and her doctor would update us on her progress and how her legs were healing. The head nurse informed her that on July 9th an ambulance would come to Glen Oaks and pick her up and transport her to Nashville. All weekend she

was so excited. Frequently, she'd ask the nurse if everything
was confirmed to make the trip to Vanderbilt. Because of
Mama's executive secretary background, she was a "check
and double-check" kind of person. Mama did not like surprises.

On Monday morning, July 9th, Mama called me crying. The ambulance service hired to transport her to Nashville did not show up at Glen Oaks. There was a conflict
with scheduling and the ambulance service did not tell Glen
Oaks till that morning. Since mama's doctor only saw patients on Mondays, the appointment had to be rescheduled
for the following Monday. Mama was heartbroken when
they told her she couldn't make her appointment. It was
like telling a little girl she couldn't go to the party. I felt so
sorry for her. I shared with her what our pastor says about
disappointments--"Disappointments are an opportunity for
an appointment with God." Maybe one more week of healing and rehab would prove to be a greater encouragement
for her next appointment. *"Oh Lord, please give her some kind
of encouragement. She's done so well. She needs a little reward."*
A few hours later she called me back. This time she wasn't
crying, but full of excitement. Her doctor had called and
ordered her stitches to be taken out at Glen Oaks. She was
so giddy! Party back on!

• • • •

Mary Lee has always had a dream. Since she was a little girl she has loved China, especially Chinese toddlers. Over the last few years she would talk about going to China and serve in an orphanage. Through lots of prayer and God miraculously intervening, she was leaving the third week of July with an organization/ministry called *Show Hope*. *Show Hope*, founded by Stephen Curtis Chapman, helps families adopt orphans. They have a facility in China called *Maria's Big House of Hope*, which is an orphanage for primarily special needs kids under the age of five. Mary Lee raised money for her trip with the help of very generous families and friends. Before she left, I wanted to be able to spend some time with her, help her pack, and take her to the airport. My baby was going to China for ten days and I just could not miss seeing her off. I knew this would mean having someone spend the night with Daddy and pulling a 24-hour shift. E.B. knew how to make a sandwich for Daddy's dinner, but I needed someone to cook the big meals…and understand food rotations! It would also mean extra money to pay a caregiver. I knew the length of time away from my duties with daddy would be very expensive. Again, all I knew to do was pray.

You know how sometimes God brings someone in your life and you know you'll be friends forever. Well, that's

my friend Susan. We started working together in the late
80's in a personnel office outside of Nashville. Just like with
Christine, when Susan and I met we loved each other instantly. Susan and I have walked through so much together
over the years and even when I decided to be a stay-at-home
mom, she and I continued to stay the best of friends. Susan
is my "has lived life" friend, so when she offers me words of
wisdom, I know to listen. I've watched her go through trials
and challenges yet continue to hang on to God and allow
Him to redeem and restore the valley years. Susan is a giver
and doesn't have a selfish bone in her body. She called me
one day and said, "I'm putting a check in the mail." Now
with my Susan there is no arguing with her. She loves to
bless and she wanted me free to have a couple of days with
Mary Lee and not have to worry about money. Her gift
more than covered my time away. After crying with great
joy and praising God, I set up E.B. to cover for me. He wanted the hours and I needed the time. I made meals ahead of
time so all he would have to do is heat them up. Praise God!
This was the best blessing, as well as an incredible witness
to Mama and Daddy how God was providing. My God can
build ramps and provide time away. He is so good. I was
also glad to have another week to prepare Daddy for my
absence.

Journal Entry | July 11th

Well today is 30 days. Only sixty more days to go before the Long Term Healthcare pays and I can be gone more. In a way time has gone by quickly, but then I think, I'm only a third of the way there. I can tell my emotions have leveled out more which is good. I'm not crying like I did. Next week is China, so I'm leaving Wednesday thru Friday evening. I'm so excited that E.B. is coming the majority of the time... and that he wants too. Lord, my prayer is for You to keep E.B., and his family all healthy, safe and at peace next week. Keep Mary Lee healthy and protected for this trip. You designed this trip Lord, and You seeded this love and compassion inside of her for China. I'm trusting You to follow through in every area and to get her there safely and back. Make her dream come true. What an amazing gift You are giving her! Thank you Lord. Oh, one more thing about the thirty days, with sixty days to go...I do need to fill up this journal so I guess let's keep going!

• • • •

As negative and worrisome as my daddy was, no doubt he was such a funny man. I would go through so many days where I'd say over and over in my head, "How did my mother do this?" Then there would be those times when he was so funny that I knew it was God saying, "*But look how unique I made him.*" In fifty-six years of marriage my mother had to be just as entertained by his silliness to balance out the negative. I'm sure he kept her laughing, just like he was making me laugh.

Journal Entry | July 12th

Daddy's funnies for the day:

—While I was taking a shower I forgot to give Daddy the house phone. It never rings, but of course, when I didn't take it to him...it rang. When I got out of the shower he said, "Jo, the phone rang...and I couldn't no more get up and get it than fly!" I laughed out loud. He thought it was funny too.

—When I scratch Daddy's back he always says the same thing, "Jo that's old hide!"

—Daddy peed a ton yesterday and last night. I was up 4 times! At 6:00 am when I stood there with him the fourth time he said, "Jo, I'm trying to set a record." I just had to laugh.

—*Daddy knows nothing about cell phones. He's even
a little intimidated by them. I was showing him how
the phone works and one of the pictures of me and Jeff.
I realized I had to go to the bathroom, so I let him hold
my phone. While I'm in the bathroom he says, "Jo, the
light went out."*
Me – "Just press one of the buttons."
Daddy – "Any letter?"
Me – "Yep."
Daddy – "Not a number?"
Me – "No, just any letter."
Daddy – "Push it now?"
Me – "Yes."
Daddy – "OK, it's back on."

*When I came out of the bathroom, he looked so in-
nocent and with a little boy face said, "I pushed 'P'."
That was the dilemma…he couldn't decide which letter
to choose.*

—*Daddy cracks me up. I asked him if he wanted to
use the urinal before I went outside to take a quick
walk. As he started going, he began talking in his
quiet, announcer, golf-commentator voice--"Billy will
now use the urinal." How does he think of this stuff?*

—*When talking to Daddy about E.B. spending the*

night next week, he said, "Well, all I need to know is
which side of the bed he wants." Then, he followed
up with, "Now Rhoda always likes to get up behind
my back." I told him we'd have to probably pay E.B.
more for that. We both had a good laugh, so I knew he
would adapt just fine.

• • • •

Fridays were the hardest days. It seemed to be the
day I wanted to cry and feel sorry for myself. I didn't feel
like talking to God, and I didn't feel like being thankful or
praising Him. *"Wow, is this really the real me? The Mary Jo*
you created, Lord?" It seemed awfully like a "rebellious Mary
Jo!" I want to be content so badly...with everything. When
I was home I couldn't look at my bed, because it made me
sad. I couldn't look at my kitchen because it made me sad. I
felt like I walked around confused. It was hard to just relax
and be content. I wanted to have a fulfilled feeling, but
instead I was anxious. There was part of me that felt obli-
gated to give out to Jeff and Mary Lee, but I felt dry. I was
serving Daddy every day, so when I was with Jeff and Mary
Lee, I was so emotionally exhausted. I also felt like time
was standing still at Daddy's house, while my family and
friends' lives continued on. I wondered if God was doing

some refining in me. I thought about the scripture in Malachi 3:3,

> *"He will sit like a refiner of silver, burning away the dross. He will purify the Levites, refining them like gold and silver, so that they may once again offer acceptable sacrifices to the Lord."*

I remembered Laurel, a spiritual mentor of mine, teaching me about how a silversmith refines silver. The whole process of firing silver is for the dross, the imperfections, to come to the surface, so the silversmith can scoop it off. I guess all of this "dross" in me was coming to the surface. It was not pretty; in fact, it was embarrassing, especially to ME! As the old *DC Talk* song says, *"I'm still a man in need of a Savior."* I so needed Jesus. I guess this was a way to make me more in the image of Christ and to be more Christ-like. It honestly felt a lot like work and even painful at times. I guess He thought I was worth it. So, when I'm more Christ-like, THEN would it be fulfilling? Was this going to be a continuous dying to me? I had a feeling the Apostle Paul would have said a big *"YES! It's daily Mary Jo!"* I thought about the end of Romans Chapter 7 when Paul also talked about how because of his flesh he did what he didn't want to do or wouldn't do what he wanted to do. He struggled with the same selfish, carnal, fleshy stuff too! His solution, as would be mine, lied in Romans 7: 24-25, which says,

"Who will rescue me from this body that is subject to
death? Thanks be to God, who delivers me through
Jesus Christ our Lord!"

I also wondered in my walk with God, would there always be a contentment battle going on inside of me? As all of the questions went through my head, it was almost comical how I taught many times in bible studies about the struggle with the spirit and the flesh. With total confidence in the power of God's Word, I would passionately teach others about crucifying the flesh and walking in the spirit--by the power of the Holy Spirit. The battle inside of me was on, but what brought me hope was my heart's desire to find peace and contentment within me. I wanted to enjoy Jesus, enjoy my family, and enjoy my life.

<u>Jesus Calling</u> | July 14th

"Keep walking with Me along the path I have chosen
for you. The journey is arduous at times, and you
are weak. Someday you will dance light-footed on the
high peaks; but for now, your walk is often plodding
and heavy. All I require of you is to take the next
step, clinging to My hand for strength and direction.

*Though the path is difficult and the scenery dull at the
moment, there are sparkling surprises just around the
bend."*

Journal Entry | July 14th

*OK, I'll stay on the path. You're right, it is dull at
times, but when Daddy is funny, it's like a little spar-
kle. It definitely feels heavy at times, like I'm carrying
the weight of keeping it together for Daddy. I still
know You are faithful God, and You are here with me.*

As difficult as I thought I had it, my cousins, Dawn
and Tammie, were hurting even more. Uncle Haywood
continued to get worse, which was so hard for them to
watch. At Glen Oaks one day, Dawn collapsed in my arms
and released a huge cry. The situation was so emotionally
draining for them and for my Aunt Betty. Uncle Haywood
really wanted to go be with the Lord. He wasn't scared or
anxious. He just wanted to go to his heavenly home. He
was so sure of it. I prayed in my heart, *"Lord, I ask you to be
merciful. If Uncle Haywood has no desire to walk, go home, think,
do anything, then would you take him home? I bind him from himself, and loose him into Your hands, Lord. Thank you Lord that he
is saved and knows where he's going. Help Aunt Betty stay strong*

spiritually and emotionally in You."

Even as I prayed daily for them, I would catch myself still consumed with me. **No weight bearing till September.** Funny how every time I heard that month it made me cry. September was so far away, yet I knew when it would finally arrive the summer would be over. I had to focus on day-to-day and not think that way.

I was so proud of Mama. I knew she hurt for me and I tried so hard not to cause her to cry. I tried to be positive around her and keep a smile on my face. I tried to tell her only the funny things Daddy would say, until he got me upset, and then I would have to tell her the not so funny moments. What was comical was her gentle nod as if to say, "Welcome to my World." In an odd way, there was something comforting about venting to the only person who understood, and there she was with two broken legs. She was way too familiar with his little sayings, the way he picked, his crazy routine, the food rotations, and so on.

One day out of the blue Daddy called me "Mama." In fact, he did it several times throughout the day, and I have to admit, I did not like it. I didn't want to take Mama's place and I sure didn't want that role. I wanted to be Mary Jo. I wanted to be Jeff's wife. I wanted to just be mama to Mary Lee and Ellen. Honestly, hearing him say "Mama" did not make me sad, but instead made me mad...at God. I tried to give sacrifices of praise daily, but like a kid, I just wanted to

be mad. My only conclusion was there was a lot of flesh-dy-
ing I needed and God knew exactly which buttons to push.
I felt selfish…I was tired…I felt lifeless…I had nothing to
look forward to. You know the most painful part? I wasn't
the Christian I thought I was. I was not the strong woman
of God I thought I was. I talked a good game and preached
to others what they should do in their particular situation
and life struggle. I felt so embarrassed. I felt like a fraud. I
felt like God had exposed how weak and powerless I was. I
thought I was a strong believer, but my mother was the one
who was the "real deal!" She displayed daily that she was
truly a woman of faith. She was walking out her faith, hanging on to God and trusting Him. I, on the other hand, was
tired and my thoughts were dry and meaningless.

Journal Entry | July 17th

Nothing has lifted. I feel exposed. Like God said,
"See…you don't have a clue what it means to love, to
serve, or to do things as unto the Lord." He's right.
So then… OK. I'm shallow, selfish and tired. I miss
my life, time with Jeff, time with Mary Lee and time
with friends. I miss freedom and variety. So now I
don't call the shots in my life. I don't control a thing.
Every day is the same except for a change in breakfast
meats. I'm not a wife first anymore. I'm not a mama
first anymore. I'm not a friend first anymore. I'm

"Mama" to my daddy and ...well, there really is not
an "and", that's just the way it is. I'm setting aside
reading Jesus Calling for a while and I'm done reading
the Word. I'll rely on worship music. I just can't read
right now. It's just empty words.

• • • •

Just when you feel you are at the end of your rope
and you are ready to throw in the towel, God will do something very sweet just to keep you going. Like a carrot dan-
gling in front of a horse, He will throw a little hope in front
of you to make you take another step forward. Simultane-
ously, He will look your way with compassion and love,
while quickly glancing at Satan saying, "BACK OFF!" At my
lowest point God sent Pastor Tom back over to the house.
Tom didn't come to socialize, but to bring communion.
The Body and the Blood...poured out for me...for as long
as I partake, I do it in remembrance of Him. I desperately
needed to be in remembrance of what Jesus did for me. I
needed my mind to focus on His sacrifice. I needed to remember who I was in Christ AND I need to remember WHO
I belonged to.

As Tom administered the elements, I closed my eyes
and had a wonderful vision. I could see myself sitting to
the right of Jesus, not as an adult, but as a little girl. Jesus

was giving me the communion and as Tom was saying the words, I could see Jesus saying them to me. It was peaceful.

By the way, the "not going to read the Word or *Jesus Calling*" thing…well, that would be like not eating anymore. No doubt, I was a starving woman.

Jesus Calling | July 18th

"I Am nearer than you think, richly present in all your moments. You are connected to Me by Love-bonds that nothing can sever. However, you may sometimes feel alone, because your union with Me is invisible. Ask Me to open your eyes, so that you can find Me everywhere."

Journal Entry | July 18th

Huge difference this morning! It's lifted…like coming out of a fog or like a dark cloud has lifted. It's like I can talk again without crying. Lord, I have felt so alone the last few days. Thank you for the prayers of the saints. Lord, I know you had the Body of Christ praying for me. Thank you. They are amazing. Their prayers have changed everything. Forgive me for being mean and disrespectful to You. I do feel like self-pity is the culprit that brings depression, anger and loneliness in my thoughts and emotions. If you would Lord, please bless each of these women abundantly.

Let me always honor them and their families.

• • • •

I really enjoyed the next few days. It felt like I was back to normal within myself. It was time to help Mary Lee pack and get ready for China. I couldn't believe it was time for her to leave. She was so excited and ready to love on some Chinese orphans. Many people would ask me, "Are you nervous about Mary Lee going to China?" Or, they would say, "I know you're scared to death about Mary Lee going." I'm not sure whether I didn't have time to think about it, or if it was God's peace, but it never crossed my mind to worry. Knowing that my daughter has loved China since she was a little girl, then seeing God open some pretty miraculous doors for her to go there, made me assume this was His doing…not mine. Since He was in charge, surely she was in good hands. If Mary Lee had shown any signs of worry or fear, then that would have bothered me, but she never batted an eye. Here was a girl who would panic when walking in a room full of people, yet getting on a huge plane and flying to the other side of the world didn't shake her. She was peaceful, excited, and ready to go.

As we left her with the Show Hope group at the airport, it just seemed like she grew. She showed such maturity. I thought how ironic it was that I had a harder time letting her grow up, than letting her go to China. I knew she would have a God-adventure for the next ten days, and since I couldn't do one thing for her while she was gone, I had to simply trust God. Yes, I could pray...but as a mother that is sometimes the hardest thing to do. You would rather have a list of things to do for them, and prefer to be on standby just in case they yell, "Mama!" And of course, if anyone should happen to mistreat your baby, the Mama bear in you has to take somebody out! But, all I had was my prayers and the prayers of family and friends. That was sufficient.

After returning home from the airport, I spent the rest of the day and evening with Jeff. For the two and a half days I was gone from Shelbyville, I didn't think very much about Mama and Daddy. I guess that was OK. I knew my mind couldn't be in two places and I wanted to be fully focused on my family. I trusted that E.B. was just fine with Daddy and if he needed me, he would call. I also left a few phone numbers of close friends if he needed them. Thankfully, all was quiet.

The day came when I had to go back on duty. Daddy was happy to see me and E.B. said things ran pretty smooth. As E.B. was leaving, he pulled me off to the side and said, "I'm exhausted...I don't see how you've been doing this every day. Mr. Billy is so great and so funny, but he requires a lot of time and attention. I just wanted you to know you're

doing a great job." Wow! I needed to hear that. I appreciated him telling me I was doing a good job, but I needed
more to hear that this job was hard. Sometimes Satan would
whisper in my ear that I was being a big baby, and to just
suck it up. There was freedom in E.B. telling me this, and
oddly, this strengthened me. In the midst of being so tired, I
needed this confirmation.

Jesus Calling | July 21st

"Rest in My Presence when you need refreshment.
Many people turn away from Me when they are ex-
hausted. They associate Me with duty and diligence,
so they try to hide from My Presence when they need a
break from work. How this saddens Me."

"Lean on, trust in, and be confident in the Lord with
all your heart and mind and do not rely on your own
insight or understanding."

Proverbs 3:5 AMP

Journal Entry | July 21st

Thank you Lord for this word today. You know how
I love this verse. It's my very favorite. I do think I've
been associating You with duty and diligence, and that
staying with Daddy is YOUR duty for me. I've felt I
have to be diligent because YOU'VE called me to this.

I'm sorry for not confidently drawing strength from
You today...and every day. Help me Lord. Praise
music and listening to the Katinas is so helpful. My
soul desperately needs it. So, it's just really hit me
that my baby, Mary Lee, is in China. Oh God, I'm so
trusting You to bless her and bring her home. I miss
her so much. Being here still brings sadness to me.
I've got to find Your peace in this and walk in content-
ment. I'm so many weeks away and I can't emotion-
ally handle this the way I have been. Help me hunger
for You and thirst for You. I have to stay filled. I have
to draw near to You. I have to abide in You. Help me
link my arm in Yours and hang on.

• • • •

It was so hard for Mama to watch her brother suffer
so much. I wondered often if the dying process was harder
on the person or the loved ones. On July 22nd, Uncle Haywood left the earth and was present with Jesus. The Lord
was so faithful. God was merciful to him and I believe He
had already settled in Aunt Betty's heart that her husband
was going home soon. My sweet mama was so sad, but
she knew beyond a shadow of a doubt that God had placed
them together at Glen Oaks. In the book of Esther it says,

"For such a time as this." God's timing can be hard to understand, and we will even disagree with it, but nevertheless, it is HIS timing not ours. As we all stood in the hallway outside Uncle Haywood's room it was peaceful, yet very sad. I watched my cousins cry like little girls who just lost their daddy. Then it hit me, "They lost their daddy." They knew they would see him again one day in heaven, but for now, they wouldn't see him anymore, or hear his voice, or endure his picking at them. I looked at my mother's face. She was so brave, yet her heart was broken. I thought about in the Word when it says in heaven there will be no more pain and no more sorrow. Sorrow is an interesting word. It is a word that is hard to describe. To understand it, it has to be experienced...similar to love. Love has to be experienced. You can teach ABOUT love, but you can't teach someone "love". It has to be caught. It has to be experienced from the one who IS love. I don't think you can teach sorrow...it also has to be experienced. It is felt deeply all the way to your very core. I realized that day, while standing in the nursing home hallway, that sorrow can be so tangible. If I had the power that day, I would have sucked out the sorrow in that place.

I had to leave to go home to a daddy I still had living, and leave my precious mother. Sometimes there is no reasoning or thoughts that make sense. Sometimes you just want to shut your brain off and just rest in knowing God

is the only one who has the answers. He knows we can't
handle all the answers. I'm good with that.

As I walked out the door of the nursing home and
drove off, the sky was filled with the biggest rainbow I had
ever seen. It was huge and the colors were as bright as
fresh paint. I pulled over to the side of the road and sent a
text message to my cousins. They both quickly replied that
they had seen it too! It brought a smile to their faces and
confirmed in their hearts, "Daddy made it home." What
an amazing God! His promises are true and His timing IS
perfect.

For the next couple of days Mama cried off and on.
Daddy wanted to see her, but he has never been very good
at comforting. He told her she was tough and she would
get through it. I knew in his own way he thought he was
encouraging her, but it wasn't a time for her to be tough.
Crying and sadness was just so uncomfortable for Daddy. I
guess that's why he did such a great job making the atmosphere light at a funeral home. There's a time to laugh and
a time to cry, and I told Mama it was good to cry. I love
Psalms 56:8, *"You keep track of all my sorrows. You have collected
all my tears in your bottle. You have recorded each one in your
book."* God bottles our tears. He truly cares about them and
knows we will have them. Crying can be so cleansing, and
grieving tears just can't be left inside. We have to get them
out, otherwise, how can God bottle them? Crying draws us

to the throne of grace so we can receive comfort in our time
of need.

> *"So let us come boldly to the throne of our gracious*
> *God. There we will receive his mercy, and we will find*
> *grace to help us when we need it."*
> *Hebrews 4:16 (NLT)*

I decided to relax on Mama's patio, before going to
the visitation. While I was talking to her on the phone,
I watched a beautiful redbird bathe in Mama's birdbath.
He was so awesome. All of the sudden, he took flight and
headed straight for me! It almost took my breath away. It
landed on the rail of the patio right in front of me. I froze
and tried to be so still. I didn't want him to go. His stay was
only a few seconds, but what a blessing it was. I told Mama
what had happened and she said, "My mother loved redbirds...maybe that was my mother?" I laughed and assured
her it was not Granny, but just a bird. We both knew, just
like seeing the rainbow, God was speaking comfort, peace,
and beauty.

Daddy couldn't go to the visitation, nor could Mama.
I had to go solo and represent our family. Uncle Haywood's
visitation was very nice. Shelbyville has always been such
a close-knit town, and seems like there's only a couple of
"degrees of separation" there. Everyone has some kind of

connection with everyone. Also, when you move away from Shelbyville, the only time you see people you grew up with is at reunions and visitations. So many people came up to me to get an update on Mama and Daddy, which was very sweet and appreciated. It was a long afternoon and evening for Dawn, Tammie, and my Aunt Betty. I knew they were worn out, but they continued to greet, love people, and receive love back.

Uncle Haywood's funeral was so sweet and the music was beautiful. Both Mama and Daddy got to be there. I handled getting daddy to the church, and Tammie made arrangements for my mother to be picked up in a van with a wheelchair lift. She even took my mother an outfit by the nursing home, which worked perfectly with the casts on her legs. She really took good care of her Aunt Rhoda. Mama was so thankful to go to the funeral and she just looked lovely. In wheeling Daddy in the sanctuary, it seemed best to park him right behind Mama at the ends of the church pews. As I looked at them, I never dreamed I would be at a funeral with both of my parents in wheelchairs. At first, I sat by Daddy, but when I saw my mother's tears, I got up and sat by her. I knew Daddy would not mind, plus he had a history of whispering very loud in church. He thought the music was too loud for his hearing aid, so he leans over in sarcasm and says, "Jo, see if they can turn that organ music up...I think she's got the pedal to the floor." I had to laugh, but my mother turned her head, which meant she heard him too. I figured I'd be safe from trouble if I sat by Mama.

It was so apparent that Uncle Haywood was loved very much. Family, friends, co-workers, and people in the community came to pay their respects and said such kind words to his family. Even though Mama knew this day was coming, it was still very difficult. Even when the mind is prepared, it seems the heart never is. It was so sweet watching people come over to Mama and tell her they had been praying for her and her legs. Shelbyville has always been full of people anointed to bless and encourage. It was a blessing to witness them do what they do best.

<u>Jesus Calling</u> | July 25th

"As you listen to birds calling to one another, hear also My Love – call to you. I speak to you continually: through sights, sounds, thoughts, impressions, scriptures. There is no limit to the variety of ways I can communicate with you. Your part is to be attentive to My messages, in whatever form they come. You can find Me not only in beauty and birdcalls, but also in tragedy and faces filled with grief. I can take the deepest sorrow and weave it into a pattern for good"

Journal Entry | July 25th

Very fitting for today. Redbirds and grief…God, You

*are in both. Help me see You in all things today…
watching the birds outside and seeing faces and voices
today at the funeral…help me, Holy Spirit, recognize
You in all things.*

I believe Uncle Haywood fulfilled this scripture:

*"No wonder my heart is glad, and I rejoice. My body
rests in safety. For you will not leave my soul among
the dead or allow your holy one to rot in the grave.
You will show me the way of life, granting me the joy
of your presence and the pleasures of living with you
forever."*

Psalm 16:9-11 (NLT)

• • • •

I missed Mary Lee so much. I thought they would
email their parents from China, or I would have at least
heard from the supervisors of the trip, but I didn't hear a
peep. I was thankful the trip was coming to a close and
she would be heading back to Chicago, then she could at
least text me before the connecting flight to Nashville. I
told Daddy how much I missed her and I hadn't heard one
word and he said, "Well, you haven't heard from Mary Lee

because she's joined the communist party!" Goodness, my
daddy could come out with the funniest and craziest stuff.

I was so ready to be at the airport and ready to see
Mary Lee. So many questions went through my mind, "Will
God call her to be a missionary in China?" I have always
loved the excitement of picking someone up at the airport.
I love the experience of standing and waiting as you look
down the long terminal, excited to see the face of the person
you're taking home. Seeing her beautiful face appear and
watching her make the walk down the terminal made me
a proud mama. What a gift from God...to be a mama. My
baby was home from China! I never thought in a million
years I would be saying that about a child I gave birth to just
a few years ago.

On the ride back to Murfreesboro, Mary Lee
shared some of her adventures. The sweetest story she
shared made me so proud. At the orphanage all the kids
were under five. Mary Lee's team had twenty people, so
when it was playtime with the kids everyone flocked to the
adorable toddlers. These were the children fun to interact
with, yet on one of the floors of the facility Mary Lee knew
there were some Chinese down-syndrome babies. These babies did not get held often by outsiders, only by the Chinese
nannies. So she and another team member decided God was
calling them to spend their time with these special babies.
Each day during "playtime", Mary Lee and her friend would

go hold the babies. I asked her if she prayed over them. She said, "Well Yeah!" (as if to say "are you kidding?") She followed up with, "Since the Chinese nannies didn't speak English, I could pray out loud over the babies." How precious... what an amazing vision!

The other story Mary Lee told me was also precious, but in a funny way. We had bought her a journal for this trip. The idea, of course, was for her to write down all her God stories. I knew this would be a stretch for Mary Lee, because she was not a journal-type person. I still hoped she would be inspired to do it. So I asked her if she wrote in it at all. Her response was, "I wrote in it for three days, then I thought...who am I writing to? Myself? God? The Journal?... so I stopped." Her journaling days started and stopped in three days, but her memories and pictures would be her treasure.

CHAPTER SIX

Learning More
and Moving Past Me

One thing had definitely become apparent the last two months…time was an idol in my life. Now more than ever before time meant so much more to me. I had been a control-freak of my time--when I do what and who I do it with. Even when God would call me to minister to someone, I would tend to think in the back of my mind, "Wait, I can't do it then…I need to do this or that time." Sometimes I would like to turn back time and not waste so much of it, or at least make it count for something. I felt like time away from Shelbyville was precious time, so I didn't want to fill it. I just wanted to hold it. Time was also sad to me. My summer was about over and there was no time with Mary Lee. I even sometimes felt like everyone has forgotten me. Even though I would still text my sisters in Christ with updates, I got fewer responses. Time was moving on and I was standing still...fixing meals and holding urinals. This made me sad. Again, I felt forgotten. I felt like God controlled my time, and well, not what I expected. Therefore, a part of me didn't want to trust God or give Him my time.

Jesus Calling | August 2nd
"Bring me the sacrifices of your time; a most precious commodity."

Journal Entry | August 2nd
Well, this is funny...sort of...sacrifice of time...time with God...time.

• • • •

"Lord, You are going to have to teach me not to be so easily offended with Daddy. I love him and he can be so enjoyable, then he can turn on a dime. I know Satan would like nothing better than to cause offense between me and Daddy. I know his world revolves so differently than mine, but I was so taken by surprise today."

So here is what happened. We went to visit Mama and she told me she had been craving Chinese eggrolls. While she and Daddy talked, I drove up the street and bought a couple of eggrolls and a couple of spring rolls. I knew Daddy would enjoy them too. When I got back to the room they "oooo'd" and "ahhhh'd" over them and sure enough, Daddy ate two of them. When we got home I asked him what he wanted for lunch. He said, "Not much Jo, those eggrolls filled me up." There was a half of a Burger King Whopper left over from the night before, so I asked if he wanted me to heat it up. He said that would be fine. I heated it up, added a few chips and brought him to the table. He ate and continued with his normal routine of going to the back bedroom for ballgames and his relaxation time. I cleaned up the kitchen and was thinking about how I would relax a bit. In a few minutes, I could hear his walker coming down the hall. It was odd and I wasn't sure what he needed. He sat down in the chair next to the closet in the den and proceeded to say, "Jo, are we going to just run out of food?" I was so shocked and I wasn't sure what he meant or what to say, but I could tell there was irritation backing his tone.

I asked, "What do you mean?" in a nice tone.

He replied, "Well, all I had was a half a burger for dinner (which I think should be called lunch)."

I replied, "You had those eggrolls and I asked what you wanted and you said not much because they filled you up?"

He shot back by saying, "Well, I'm afraid you're going to just wait around till we don't have anything to eat. There's no planning!"

OK, at this point I am really caught off-guard and I am trying to understand his thinking and point of view. Since June 6th, he had not missed a beat in meals. He had a meat and two vegetables with a salad or slaw every day. Then it dawned on me...I served him a burger at lunch! A burger was NOT a lunch or dinner food...it was for supper only! I had thrown him completely off course. I seriously had rocked his world and he was genuinely ticked at me.

I tried in a nice way to explain that I thought he would enjoy the half of burger, since he said he wasn't very hungry. It just was not sticking, in fact; he wasn't even listening to my words. Daddy continued to insult his meals and lack of variety and the possibility of running out of food. I'm not sure if it was my fatigue or if I decided I wasn't going to accept his criticism or correction, but I snapped slightly. I kept my tone calm, but increased to a sterner voice. I said, "Daddy, I have a whole refrigerator and freezer full of food. I asked you if the half burger was fine for lunch and you said it was fine. And since I've gotten here you haven't missed a meal!"

This didn't help at all. He snapped right back, "Now wait a minute, I don't understand why you have to talk ugly to me. I know I haven't missed a meal. You're blowing this out of proportion. I'm just making conversation."

Seriously, this was his idea of conversation? "OK Daddy, you tell me some dinners you want and I'll write them down and get the food and we'll have them." I tried so hard to act like it was fine and I really wanted to know what meals he was missing out on. What I wanted to say was, "Hey, in this whole scenario YOU are the only one whose schedule has not changed. You haven't been inconvenienced once, yet you are on your soapbox because in your opinion a burger was served at the wrong time of day!" But in my heart I was praying, *"God, please help me stay calm...please help me be cool...please help me understand."*

He started telling me lunches he wanted and I wrote them down. Some were already in the rotation, but I didn't say a word. He followed up with, "Jo, don't be so touchy... I'm easy to please." WHAT! SERIOUSLY! *"Lord Jesus, help me!"*

Jesus Calling | August 3rd

"Watch your words diligently. Words have such great power to bless or wound. When you speak carelessly or negatively, you damage others as well as yourself. I have trained you to pray – 'Help me, Holy Spirit.' As positive speech patterns replace your negative ones, the increase in your joy will amaze you."

"My dear brothers, take note of this: Everyone should
be quick to listen, slow to speak and slow to become
angry."

James 1:19 (NLT)

It is interesting in Romans 8, Paul talks about walking in the flesh versus the spirit. When I walk in the flesh,
I'm hostile to God, and when I walk in the spirit, I'm at
peace with God. I didn't want to be hostile with God, but
I realized that I was. As I was offended, tired, selfish, or
missing home, I could tell it made me mad at God. This was
definitely not productive or sensible. *"Forgive me, Lord. I need*
peace more than anything. So help me walk in the spirit and not
the flesh. Holy Spirit, help me decrease so you can increase."
I started to pick up on the fact that Daddy could sit
and think up negative, unrealistic thoughts. He could stir
himself up in a frenzy in his head, till it just had to come
out, which I was obviously the closest target. I shared the
incident with Mama and she just shook her head and said,
"Honey, I'm sorry. You're doing a great job." She understood his mood swings and it was like a weird new connection for us. I now understood what she had gone through
for years, and therefore, she could encourage me in my
season of caregiving.
Over the last several years, I remembered praying and asking God to take Daddy home to heaven before

Mama. I wanted her to have some years to live...really enjoy life...maybe travel. She now had two broken legs and was living in a nursing home. I felt like Satan was mocking my prayers. I was tired and drained of joy. Because of my frustration, when Daddy would compliment me, he now seemed so insincere. I even thought maybe his compliments were only to keep things the way he wanted them. I loved my Daddy, but I needed more and more of God's perspective. I needed God's filling of a fresh love for Daddy. I needed to look past the funnies, the picking, the corrections...and just love him. *"I forgive Daddy, Lord...I forgive him."*

Journal Entry | August 5th

I haven't wanted to talk. I can't seem to get on top of this situation. I'll have a good day...then several depressing days. Even when I go home, it doesn't feel familiar. I feel paralyzed and misplaced. Jeff is so down too. He feels neglected as a husband. Sometimes I feel offended with him, and then I feel sorry for him. This is just screwing us up. God, are you setting us up to fail? It's not getting better. I'm worse...I'm lost. I'm frustrated and sometimes extremely sad. I know as your child I should be positive, grateful, thankful, joyful, trusting, and kind. Hey, if these traits are in me, please bring them up! If they are not in me, then this would be the ultimate sadness. Lord, please create

them in me quickly. I'm so afraid that I'm closer to the
emotion of "hating" than I am to "loving." If hating
is at one end and loving is at the extreme other end,
where exactly am I on this scale?

As I wrote and poured my heart out to God, I also told Him, *"Lord, I feel like You've stolen my life from me."* When I said it to Him, it felt so strong that this could be the root of my selfish anger. In my heart, He whispered, ***"Then lay it down, so I can give it back."***

It is amazing how when you have walked through a new situation, you tend to question who you are. I found myself asking "Who am I?" How do I lay down my life and plans and stay grounded in who I am? How do I lean into this situation and allow this opportunity to really discover myself in Jesus, my personality, my character, and my identity? And if this was a God-test, I certainly wanted to pass it. I wanted the reward of doing this so God was honored and He could count on me to serve Him with joy and a good attitude.

On the other hand, in the back of my mind I was thinking, "If I always have a good attitude and I'm always joyful, then God's going to keep me here longer and also, Mama and Daddy will want me to stay longer." Whew, I was mentally wearing myself out, wondering if I could handle the pressure and trying to answer questions that couldn't be answered. Some of my questions were:

"When can I go home?"

"When is this coming to an end?"

"What am I missing out on?"

I felt very shallow and that there should be more to me…more character, more Christ-like qualities, more commitment to Jesus. *"Lord, don't let me forget who I am…and whose I am."*

Over the next few days, God really spoke to me about time. I realized that I couldn't let my emotions be controlled by time. I had to trust God with my time, and walk in the freedom of being joyful. I wanted the freedom to show mercy to Daddy and the freedom to walk in love. I also realized I had to make a conscience decision to make Jesus Lord over my time. As long as I was lord over my time, I was missing out on good things, but if I honored God with my time, He would bring reward.

• • • •

Jesus Calling | August 8th

"The best response is a heart overflowing with gratitude."

Journal Entry | August 8th

*Lord, it has taken a while, but I'm learning this is the
key to Your heart. Just like I enjoy my girls being
grateful and thoughtful with me, how much more do
You love it when I'm that way with You?*

*"Therefore everyone who hears these words of mine
and puts them into practice is like a wise man who
built his house on the rock. The rain came down, the
streams rose, and the winds blew and beat against that
house; yet it did not fall, because it had its foundation
on the rock."*

Matthew 7:24-25 (NLT)

Even though leaving Murfreesboro was still hard, I
was not depressed or mad about it anymore. It was just a
reality. I had also decided it was OK to not feel guilty about
not wanting to leave my home. The fact was I wanted to be
home...I wanted to be with Jeff in our own bed at night...
I wanted more time with Mary Lee. It was OK to say it,
because these were the facts. The truth was I was not lord
over my time...Jesus was. I was not in charge... God was. I
didn't know the plan and what the next two to three months
looked like...but God did. And I was OK with that. I would
continue with my assignment. My "I will" proclamation
was based on Psalm 9:1-2:

"I will thank you Lord, with all my heart
I will tell of all the marvelous things you have done.
I will be filled with joy because of you.
I will sing praises to your name O Most High.
I will thank you, tell, be filled and sing!
I will."

Feelings are a wonderful thing, but they sure can dictate the day. With my change of attitude came a sweeter love for my daddy. I tried to do a better job at being less sensitive to his picking, and to simply laugh instead. Every night for the last two months, when I would hold the urinal for Daddy in the wee hours of the night, he would repeat the same routine, "Jo, am I going?" I replied, "Yep, you're going." In a few seconds, "Jo, am I done?" I replied, "Yep, you're done." Or sometimes it would be a "Yep...oh wait... not yet...OK now you're done." When he WAS finally through, he thought it was funny to ask, "Jo, how many CC's?" I made the mistake one time of telling him that urinals measure in CC's. So, instead of just taking that bit of information then letting it go, he thought it was so hilarious to ask me the CC's. Over and over again he asked about checking the CC's for the fun of it. As I would help him back to bed, then turn to leave the room to pour out the urinal, I would get the same question, "Jo, how many CC's?" He really didn't want to know...he just got a kick out of asking.

It was the same as the "get me my razor, Joe Frazier." Every day for two months, we did this routine. If this book could contain it, I could share many more lines throughout the day. I began to wonder who the parrot really was...me or Daddy. At least I was more content. He liked it, it entertained him, and it made him laugh. So, I had to tell myself, "Lighten up Mary Jo, and roll with it." When you stop fighting the current, it is easier to swim!

CHAPTER SEVEN

"I Want My Mommy"

G reat news! We found out that mama could come home at the end of August and she would be able to complete her rehab at home. Insurance would pay for someone to come three days a week to work with her. This was such wonderful news! But, why was I scared and full of anxiety? I had just gotten Daddy figured out, or maybe I just had gotten ME figured out...either way, how was this going to work? And what about E.B.? That relationship worked for Daddy, but Mama would not have another man in the house, especially taking care of her. So the first change would be to switch caregivers.

The second change was me becoming a caregiver
for two people instead of one. Daddy's walking ability had
been declining over the last few weeks. Some mornings his
hip would hurt him so bad, that I would have to roll him
in the wheelchair for breakfast. When Mama came home, I
would officially have one patient using a walker/wheelchair
combo, and the other completely non-weight bearing for another month minimum. Yes, we would have dueling wheelchairs.

My sweet mama told me, "Now honey, I won't be
any trouble because I'm self-sufficient." OK, I think she had
forgotten that she was having 24-hour nursing care at Glen
Oaks. How do you say, "No, my precious mother, you are
not really self-sufficient. Someone makes, brings and cleans
up your food. Someone cleans your potty chair. Someone
helps you with your sponge baths, etc." All of the sudden I
had that feeling of being trapped again. No freedom. But I
couldn't look at things that way. My head said I would be
hearing all day and all night long "Jo?...Honey?...Jo?...Hon-
ey?" My spirit and my heart said simply to trust God. One
day at a time was the only way to view this. Just as God had
taught me how to care for Daddy, He would show me how
to care for Mama too.

I missed her and I knew Daddy missed her too.
Throwing her in the mix could actually be fun! Well, at least
interesting. But we were a few weeks away, so time would
tell.

• • • •

A highlight of the summer was my 30-year class
reunion. It's funny how things work out. I was already
in Shelbyville! I have to say, I loved going to high school
in Shelbyville. I had many good friends and lots of good
memories. Of course, reunions can make you nervous too.
I missed my twentieth reunion, so I had mixed emotions
about going to this one. E.B. agreed to stay a little later than
usual and Daddy was very excited I was going. He loved
my old friends and they loved him. He told me, "Now Jo,
I'll need a full report tomorrow." It was nice to dress up
and put on some makeup, knowing I was going out for the
evening. Plus, it felt like a date because Jeff was picking me
up. I was hoping for an evening of laughter and joy.

And sure enough, the reunion was a blast! Seeing
old friends and actually making new friends with the ones
I didn't know very well thirty years ago. God also sent me
several friends to share their personal experiences of taking care of their parents. Most of the stories I heard were
worse than mine, which humbled me. Their testimonies
and encouragement brought me strength and refreshment.
It was like having kindred spirits or perhaps realizing you
were now a member of a club you didn't know existed before. These people were like heroes to me. *"Please bless them,
Lord."*

The next morning, I shared with Daddy who I saw at the reunion. He wanted all the details and it was fun for him to try to remember my old high school friends. The day started out very well, but for some reason he was full of himself. Every facial expression I made he would mimmick, which was odd because I wasn't aware I was making one. Everything I said he would parrot. If I casually said, "OK" or "alright", he would parrot it back in a mocking voice. It felt like one of those kids' games where the five-year-old repeats everything his older sibling says…right down to the last syllable. I was so weary I felt my jaw tensing. He was a good Daddy and I know he loved and appreciated me, but seriously…*is he five?* Mama must have really loved him, because this was so tiring and frankly--offensive.

I finally told him that he watched my face way too closely and that he exaggerated. I was honest and told him this behavior made me feel so uncomfortable. This silenced him and he pouted…until suppertime, then a Burger King Whopper brought him out of it.

● ● ● ●

Journal Entry | August 13th

Jeff reminded me of something and I had a revelation. He said I was doing the right thing. That I was

*sowing sacrifice now and would reap peace of mind
and no regrets when my parents are gone. He shared
how so many people wish they had done more and have
regrets when a parent passes. Another revelation that
I realized was I sometimes treat my Heavenly Father
like my earthly father. When I feel God has not been
fair to me, I stop talking to Him, just like I do with my
daddy. Earthly fathers can be offensive and rude one
minute, then kind and loving the next. But God isn't
like this. He never changes. He remains the same. I
can trust Him.*

Jesus Calling | August 15th

*"Talk to Me about everything. When things go
'wrong' you tend to react as if you're being punished.
Instead of this negative response, try to view difficul-
ties as blessings in disguise."*

Journal Entry | August 15th

*This nailed me, Lord. I do feel like You're punishing
me, and I feel I respond negative every time. So, You
want me to view this as blessings in disguise? OK...
Help! I don't know how, but I'm willing. Help me see
You are blessing me and not being mean to me.*

I was so blessed to have E.B. stay with Daddy, but now things were going to change. With Mama coming home, we had to get a female caregiver. In less than a month, we would have more caregivers coming in the house because long-term healthcare insurance would start paying the expenses. It was a weird feeling to look forward to the 90-day payout ending, and to also feel territorial about my parents' house. I didn't want just anyone coming in my house...oh wait, Mama and Daddy's house. I didn't want Daddy uncomfortable. I knew having female caregivers were OK with him, because he was so use to female nurses, plus he was not modest at all. I just wanted a smooth transition. I believed as E.B. made his exit, not only would he understand, but God would find him another person to care for. He had been a blessing.

During this time I felt cold symptoms coming on, which made me feel totally drained. As tired as I was it was Friday night, so I wanted to be with Jeff and see some friends. Jeff scheduled a dinner with Cindy, Kelly and three other couples. As we met at the restaurant I knew my social abilities were going to be sad. I just didn't want to talk...actually I wanted to curl up in a corner and cry. My nose was red from blowing and sniffing, so I wasn't looking too pretty either. When you look like that, sweet friends will tend to say, "You OK?" or "Mary Jo, what's wrong?" I couldn't answer those questions at the moment. My spiritual, physical, and emotional immune system was shot and tears were at the surface-- ready to burst through!

As we walked in the restaurant I spotted Cindy and Kelly. Cindy walked up and gave me a card, so I asked if I should open it. She said it was up to me. I had never been good at waiting to open cards or gifts, so I opened it up immediately. Cindy, Lisa and Tracie bought me a 90-minute massage gift certificate. OK, first of all what an awesome gift...I love massages! But, that is not what got to me. These girls have been my friends since high school. Every year for the past eight years, we have come together for a weekend at Tracie's in Atlanta, to relax, eat and laugh. Tammy, the fifth of the group, also got a certificate too. She was going through an emotional time helping a friend cope with the lost of a child. The five of us have gone from being "partners in crime" in our high school days, to sisters-in-Christ.

Although this was a great gift, it seemed like when I opened the envelope I opened an overwhelming love I can't explain. It washed over me and broke the barrier that was holding back the tears. I just lost it. Poor Cindy, not being one for emotion and tears said, "Awe Mary, if I had known it would make you cry, I would have told you to wait."

The feeling of love from my dear girlfriends felt so good, yet so humbling. They were thinking about me. I wasn't forgotten. In the words of Sally Fields, "They like me...they really like me." I made trips back and forth to the bathroom, blowing my nose and trying to stop crying, but there was nothing I could do about looking like Rudolph the Red Nose Reindeer. As we ate dinner I don't think I said but a few words. We were a party of ten, yet it could have easily been a party of nine, because I had checked-out socially. I was caught up in my thoughts and blessed beyond words. I don't remember even eating. It was a moment of tangible love I will never forget.

• • • •

One of the decisions I made in my heart was when Mama came home, she would be in charge again! I had to remember that this was her home and I wanted her to feel like she called the shots, and I was there to serve. I also knew because my mother was the ultimate planner, that she would have specific plans. The first plan of action was rearranging the house to make the living room into a bed-room. This room had to be rehab and wheelchair friendly. Her nursing home representative actually had to approve the home layout. My daddy hated change and moving things around, but I had to convince him that if we did not rearrange, then Mama could not come home. He quickly adapted to the change. I turned their large living room into a bedroom. After I moved the sofa, chairs and rolled up rugs against the walls, I scooted one of the bedroom twin beds and two nightstands in the living room space. Thank good-ness for all of the times I had watched remodeling shows on

HGTV!

As I worked on remodeling the house, the more excited I felt about Mama coming home. I wanted to make it functional, yet pretty too. I wanted that part of the show where they kept their eyes closed, and then the show says, "OK, open your eyes!" Then the recipients are shocked with pure joy at the beauty of the room. OK…the HGTV response was a little out of reach, but I wanted to make Mama proud and for her to feel wanted and to definitely feel at home.

During our strategic planning at the nursing home one day, I spoke very honest with Mama about how it was not going to be as easy as she thought. The questionable "self-sufficiency" and how coordinating two wheelchairs in the house would be a challenge. I diplomatically vented my fears to her thinking she would immediately understand, but I'll never forget her response. Tears welled up in her eyes as she said, "But, I want to come home." Oh my goodness! It broke my heart hearing those words and seeing her little girl face. I calmly and sweetly said, "Mama, I want you to come home, and it is going to be perfect." Her face went from sad to happy.

For a couple of days I moved, rearranged and set up furniture in her new bedroom. Jeff added his engineer touch and ideas on furniture arrangement which made it perfect. I did the best I could to make the room look complete and

welcoming, so I added flowers arrangements. I wanted
the room to say, "Welcome home! I've missed you!" When
she and her physical therapist came to the house, I was so
excited. Although it wasn't Mama's actual "move in" day,
she was required to be there. I actually had the mini HGTV
moment when she came through the door in her wheelchair.
She was so excited to see her new room and her home. The
last time she had been home was June 6th. Just like I had
experienced with my house, I knew she missed the smells
of her home, the warmth of her bed, and the routine of her
days. For a moment I didn't care about me going home to
Murfreesboro. I was overjoyed that she was coming home
and I would get to witness it.

We were down to one week away from Mama's
homecoming, which was so exciting and yet, made me a bit
nervous. I was ready for Mama to be in charge, and for God
to send her the perfect new caregivers. I knew they would
have to be able to take directions, because Mama was a great
delegator...or maybe more like a really, sweet, drill sergeant.
As the new caregivers started, so would a new schedule. I
had been used to living the majority of time with daddy,
so I wasn't sure what the new phase would look like. I had
learned that some things could be planned or figured out,
but other times had to simply unfold. I was counting on the
details to fall into place.

It dawned on me that I was not coming to "the end"

of something, but rather "the beginning" of something. I
didn't know whether to be excited or scared! I decided to
hang on to Jesus and ride it out. My gut feeling said I was
about to be busier, but I also knew having Mama home was
a good thing. She would not call me "Mama" or be a "parrot," so that was exciting. Oh wait, that meant she would get
the "attention" from Daddy instead of me. Hmmm...I hated
that...or did I? These were my parents and I grew up with
them, but being with them at my age was like never having
lived with them before. I knew this was going to be comical!

• • • •

Mama was home!!! Praise God! She was so excited,
but I couldn't tell if she was nervous too. Her nurses were
so sad to see her leave Glen Oaks. They had gotten to know
a special and amazing woman over the last three months.
They watched her exercise like a 25-year-old and they had
been on the receiving end of her positive attitude and encouraging words. So sad for them, but I realized I was the
next beneficiary.

The first couple of days she was home, reminded me
of how I reacted when I would go back to Murfreesboro for
my short visits. I was very disconnected and now so was
she. She loved her new bedroom and was thankful to be
home, but she finally said to me, "Honey, I just can't seem
to think." I told her I understood and I shared how I expe-

rienced those same feelings. I have to admit, it was nice not
to have to load Daddy up in the car and drive to the nursing
home. He could now see her anytime and that made him
very happy. There was a sweetness about walking into the
living room and there she was! I felt such a peace, and a
sense of normalcy returning. I was not home yet, but Mama
was, and that was an amazing feeling.

Mama also soon realized that her "needs" were more
than she had thought, and she was NOT self-sufficient. For a
self-sufficient kind of woman to not be sufficient in her own
home was humbling for her…almost embarrassing in a way.
I tried to make it humorous.

"Now Honey, I can give myself a sponge bath; you
don't have to help," she would state.

I'd reply, "Who'll get the washcloth, water and
soap…then pour the water out when you're finished?"

She would say, "Well, I guess you will."

She would then say, "Now Honey, I can dress myself."

I would reply, "Who will wash your dirty clothes, so
they'll be all clean for you?"

She would sheepishly say, "Well, I guess you will."
After we did this sort of thing a couple of times, it went from
laughing to her little girl face saying, "Oh Honey, I'm sorry
you're having to take care of me too." I reassured her that
she was a breeze compared to her husband! She laughed

again.

My mother was definitely a different eater than my Daddy. Mama could eat a cold leftover burger for breakfast and scrambled eggs and toast for supper. She was easy to please. She had lost about twenty pounds and gained some strong muscle tone over the last three months. She looked about 10 years younger! To watch this woman exercise three times a day and give it 100% was very cool. She would push and challenge herself. Daddy would stroll through the living room at times and always say, "Mama, please be careful...you're making me nervous." She would say, "Billy, I'm fine. This is just what I have to do, so go sit down!" He would say, "Well, don't push too hard and hurt yourself."

My mother knew how to push safely and how to be consistent, which was what she had to do. The results were amazing. I was so proud of her, as was her Home Health Physical Therapist, Mike. God sent her a wonderful, Christian man, who meshed with Mama perfectly for her personality. He was a tough coach, yet a gentle spirit and an encourager. Mike loved Mama's energy, capabilities, and focus. They were a good team. I knew it wouldn't be long till she would be walking again.

Even though the plan was coming together and I was caring for two, things seemed to change in me. For some reason, I fell into task mode...almost mechanical.

<u>Jesus Calling</u> | August 27th

"You have to repeat so many tasks day after day. This monotony can dull your thinking until your mind slips into neutral."

• • • •

Journal Entry | September 2nd

So having Mama home has been good. She's settling in. I'm having a tough time with joy. It's like I'm just going through the motions. I'm doing the task at hand, but it's mechanical...like I'm doing a job, instead of doing all of this as a loving daughter. And I'm not offended. I'm just sad...kind of empty feeling. It's like I'll never be home. I know it's not true, but it feels like it will never come. I'm sorry I haven't trusted or even fellowshipped with You, Lord. I'm not sure why. Maybe, I'm afraid to receive and walk in joy. Maybe, I do not totally trust this path to You. I do love you God, but can I trust you? I still find myself protecting my emotions. I feel like I show little emotion with Mama and Daddy. I say "you're welcome", when they say "thank you", but I don't dwell in the moment. I don't want to live in that place. I don't know why.

*I want to be Mama's encourager and cheerleader. I
really do. I want her to know I'm proud of her. I think
what gets me the most is the date. It's September
2nd... almost three months I've lived here---summer
gone. Time gone. I want to learn how to enjoy my
time no matter where I am or what situation I'm in.
To be in You and You in me. To praise You and thank
You for my weaknesses. To anticipate a miracle daily
and to see life through You. I have so much to learn.
Please be patient with me, Lord.*

September 10th is around the corner, so decisions
had to be made. Eighteen hours a day could be covered by
caregivers, but the remaining six would not. So how do I
cover this? There was really only one option. I decided I
would leave my house at 5:00 am and start my shift at 6:00
am, then leave at 12:00 noon. The two caregivers would
work back to back for 9-hour shifts each. Of course, this
meant I continued to cook the big meals, breakfast and
lunch, but no clean up, so I was off until 6:00 am the next
morning. I would have to resort to my college days of waking up, brushing my teeth, throwing on sweats, putting on a
cap, and then heading out the door. I figured if my college
professors didn't mind thirty years ago, then Mama and
Daddy wouldn't care either.

My husband did decide to make one request. He

wanted me home for the weekends. So the weekend caregivers would have to work 12-hour shifts and Mama and
Daddy would have to pay the overage. Jeff had been a very
patient and kind man; this wasn't asking too much and I
knew Mama would understand. When I shared with her
about not working on the weekends, she said, "I need to
give you money." I told her, "I don't want money, I want
my time." I realized that "time" should not be coveted or
an idol. Nor should time be a means of selfishness, but
time was a precious gift and it should not be wasted. Time
should be treasured and cherished…whether it was alone
time with God or time with family or time with friends. I
needed to do a better job of not wasting time. Mama agreed
to the terms peacefully.

• • • •

On September 7th, Mama's left leg had three weeks
healing over the right leg which meant the time had come
to stand on this left leg. She was excited and scared at the
same time. She could bend this leg to a 90-degree angle with
no problem, plus she had strength. She could pull and flex
like a gymnast, but standing was really the goal. She had
worked so hard and respected her legs. She was consistent,
maintained an exceptional attitude, and was very obedient
to her doctor's orders. *"Lord, please let there be no pain."* I'm
not sure who was more excited, me, Mama, or Mike the PT!

Deep down, Daddy was excited, but because he was a worrier, he was afraid of...well, he didn't really know what he was afraid of.

I was ready with my cell phone to video the moment. She had prepared herself for some pain, yet knew she had experienced the worst pain already. I watched her take some deep breaths and focus on the moment. With Mike helping with balance and Mama holding to her walker--she slowly stood up! SHE DID IT! Mama stood on her left foot! NO PAIN! PRAISE GOD! We were all excited and so thankful. Even though she would still spend a majority of the time in her wheelchair for three more weeks, this was a great start. Mike showed her how to take small steps with the walker, while she continued to stay non-weight bearing on the right leg.

Daddy was so proud of her, even though seeing her standing made him a nervous wreck. Yes, he was a champion worrier, yet he loved her so much and didn't want her to hurt. I was seeing the light at the end of the tunnel, not just for myself, but seeing Mama back to normal...wait, no not back to normal, she was better. She had a new strength, a new faith in God and an even greater positive outlook on life. She was great before, but now she was an inspiration. *"God, I want to be just like her."* I knew as I moved forward to the next phase of this journey, I wanted to be better too. I wanted to be powerful instead of pitiful.

Journal Entry | September 10th

*Day 90! Long-term healthcare starts! I can't believe
it's here. Lord Jesus, I have been here over 3 months!
Sometimes I have so many emotions about this whole
thing…thankfulness, anger, peace, sadness, hope,
disappointment, etc. A new shift starts, so if all goes
as planned, I'll be in my bed tomorrow night, which
will be a wonderful thing. You'll still have to help me,
Lord, in this next phase and get me up in the mornings. It should be interesting, but I definitely know I
can do ALL things through You! I pray the caregivers
are perfect for Mama and Daddy.*

Leaving both Mama and Daddy felt odd, yet peaceful. The drive back to Murfreesboro started a new phase. In
fact, the drive back included packing my bags. It was weird
gathering all my stuff and loading it in the car. It felt like the
day I moved out for college. My stuff I had at their house for
a few months was now going back in my drawers and back
in my closet. I could not wait to be home. Driving home
was joyful and I was very thankful. The three months taking
care of Daddy was worth this feeling of knowing I was going
home. When I walked in the kitchen there stood Jeff and
Mary Lee with their arms literally stretched out. There was
a beautiful arrangement of flowers on the table and a sign
that said, "Welcome Home." I fell in their arms and cried as

I said, "I'm so glad to be home."

Sleeping in my bed was so wonderful. I felt anxious and emotionally geared up, so I didn't sleep very much. I suspect I was waiting on someone to need help with a urinal! It's funny how the body remembers times to be awake. Nevertheless, I felt rested. Just sleeping next to Jeff was peaceful and secure. Thank you, Lord.

CHAPTER EIGHT

Seeing Him In Spite of Me

One of the things I missed when Sundays rolled around was going to my church, World Outreach Church. Even though I could watch Pastor Allen on television on Sunday mornings, it just wasn't the same. I definitely took it for granted. My first Sunday back, a guest was speaking for the morning services, but also the Sunday night too. Jeff and I decided to double up and go to both. That night a big crowd filled the sanctuary, and everyone was excited. A dear and old friend came up to me and asked about Mama and Daddy. I briefly shared and gave her an update, and then she left to find a seat. Before I sat down, the lady behind me tapped me on the shoulder and said, "Excuse me, I didn't mean to ease drop on your conversation with your friend, but did I hear you say, you've been taking care of your parents?" I said, "Yes, I have." Tears welled up in her eyes, as she had a difficult time responding back. I immediately leaned over my seat and grabbed her hands and held them tight. I waited for her to speak.

After a few seconds she said, "My father-in-law just died, but for the last year I've been his caregiver." Tears started falling down her cheeks as she continued, "I heard you say how hard it's been, but God has helped you through it. You look so full of joy, yet you've had to change your life to help them. I just want to ask you…did you ever feel guilty for not wanting to always be there?"

Wow, first I was floored by the fact that this woman saw "joy" on me. OK, that was most definitely a God-thing. Secondly, God orchestrated this whole seating arrangement so she could hear me share with my friend. The woman had lost her father-in-law, so in reality, she was no longer a caregiver, yet she was still carrying emotions of guilt…and probably many more difficult feelings.

As I continued to hold her hands tightly, I smiled and said, "Oh yes, I've run the gamut of emotions. I've felt mad about having to do it, and then guilty for feeling that way… and I have wonderful parents!"

She smiled back and said, "Thank you for telling me

that. I loved my father-in-law so much. He was a precious man. He lived with my husband and me this last year and I just basically put my life on hold to take care of him. His wife died years ago, so it's like he clung to me, maybe out of missing her. He just required a lot of attention, and well, sometimes I was just exhausted. My husband and I haven't been able to do anything together for a long time. Satan has made me feel so guilty. I hear in my head sometimes 'you didn't do a good enough job' and 'you're a bad person for not wanting to serve him.' And you felt the same way too?"

It was like relief and peace was washing over her, because there was someone else who felt those things too. I just said, "Sister, you have no idea. It's OK and you'll be fine. Just listen, cling, and let God love on YOU for a while."

Then she said, "I want the joy you have and to be able to move forward and be able to let it go. I want to enjoy my life as a couple again."

I got as close as I could to her and prayed for her. I don't remember what I prayed, but I knew God brought us together. He was mindful of us as His daughters and He cared about us moving to the next phase in our lives. He wasn't mad at us for our wishy-washy feelings throughout our caregiving. He never left our sides as we served. He was our strength, our helper, our comforter and our God in every way.

I never saw this woman again, and I don't remem-

ber her name, but I'll never forget her. I was her answered
prayer and she was mine. She was a source of refreshment
to me. She made me realize I now had a testimony. She
made me realize there were lots of caregivers out there with
bundles of emotions to deal with, and some emotions they
haven't dealt with. Whether they are taking care of parents,
in-laws, grandparents, etc., the struggles emotionally can be
the same. I thought the purpose of the evening was to be
inspired by the guest speaker, but my inspiration and the
purpose of the night was a divine appointment with a sister-
in-Christ in the seat behind me. It was the perfect night out.

• • • •

At the end of September, Mama stood on both legs.
Woo Hoo! She looked like a baby giraffe learning to walk.
She was adorable. After a few days, she ditched the wheelchair and stuck with the walker. There was no stopping
her now! For four weeks I continued my six-hour shift with
weekends off. The caregivers continued to do a great job,
but I knew it would not be long until my mother would
want everybody (including me) out of her house. But she
was patient. The four weeks of my morning shift ended up
being pretty entertaining. We three would sit at the kitchen
table and I would just listen to their conversations. One
morning they had a debate on whose wheels were bigger on
their walkers. Another morning, they got into the familiar

discussion of who looked best in their casket at the funeral
home. They each gave their top three best, then their top
two worst. Fascinating! Listening to them at six o'clock in
the morning made me realize they were very unique parents.
It dawned on me, for the whole time I stayed with Daddy,
he never woke up in a bad mood. He woke up every morning talking, joking, making silly faces, picking or making
goofy noises, but he was never mad. My mother would say,
"Your father is a morning person, but I like to just be quiet
first thing in the morning." So, I guess I was like my mother.
All those mornings he was talking and talking, and I would
just listen...well, sometimes I would fake listen. He enjoyed
doing all the talking, because it was what he was used to, so
again, his routine stayed the same socially too. Now with
Mama at home, I could let her respond and watch her roll
her eyes at his tacky, yet funny comments. My goodness...
they had been doing this song and dance for years and years.

After breakfast one morning, I walked up the driveway to get Daddy's newspaper. That trip was all of twenty-
five seconds. When I walked back in the kitchen, Daddy was
sitting on the floor! Mama was standing beside him, shaking
her head saying, "I don't know what happened." *OK, how
did he get in the floor just within seconds?* "Daddy, what happened?"

He said, "I don't know, Jo. I was trying to get up and
just slid down in the floor." Mama was standing there want-

ing to help, but knowing there was not one thing she can do. So, we went through the not so pretty procedure of trying to get him back in the chair. Daddy cooperated very well, so he was up in just a few minutes. This experience brought up a very important conversation between me and Mama. "Now Mama, you are to never, ever try to help Daddy up! If he pulled you down you could reinjure your legs and do some terrible damage." She half listened to me and said, "Oh, I know how much I can do and not do."

OK, she did not get it at all. "Mama! Look at me. If you fall you would be back at Glen Oaks again. Do you want to do that? AND, I am not going through this again." I laughed saying that final line, but actually, I was pretty serious. She heard this time and said, "You're right Honey, I promise I won't try to get him up. I'll call a neighbor or the police if I have to."

"Lord, please make her keep her promise!"

• • • •

At the end of October, Jeff and I planned a vacation to the beach…just the two of us. At the first of November, I scheduled my annual high school girl's trip to Tracie's in Atlanta. We also made the decision to not have our annual Thanksgiving at our house, but instead our family would fly to Colorado Springs and have Thanksgiving with Ellen and Joe. Ellen was a great cook, so she wanted to handle all the cooking. What? No cooking for me? Praise the Lord!!! Three trips in place, which meant by the end of October my six-hour shift would be over.

So the question was could Mama and Daddy handle the six hours on their own? By the end of October, Mama was getting around great, but Daddy seemed to need his wheelchair more. After a brainstorm meeting with Mama, she and I decided the six hours of "no care giving" time would be from three o'clock in the afternoon until nine o'clock at night. Daddy was going to be in the back bedroom anyway, so most of those hours would be their relaxing time. Mama and I enforced the best we could that he was limited to getting up and down during this time frame. Since supper was a sandwich or salad, Mama assured me she could handle it. I was a bit nervous, but she wanted the six hours without caregivers so badly. She was actually excited about it. It was like the next step to freedom and independence for her. Go Mama! All in all, they did pretty good, although each day Daddy continued to not feel good.

The last week of October, Jeff and I headed to Florida to spend a week on the beach. No words could describe how excited I was to go on this trip. My husband, the warm weather, the beach, the seafood...I was thrilled! Jeff had been working so hard and I knew he needed this trip as much as I did. Plus, he and I needed to reconnect with each other. Right before we left, a huge account opportunity surfaced with his job. I was used to Jeff having to do a little work while on vacation, but this seemed to be more than a few minutes here and there. When we reached our condo and opened the door, we were very pleased. The condo was perfect, except for one thing-- he couldn't get internet to work. This began a 48-hour ordeal of frustration, anger, and panic for Jeff. Several times he would say, "We may not be able to stay. If I can't get internet and my computer to connect we will have to go home. I have to be able to work here."

OK, this was not what I wanted to hear. I had been waiting on this trip. We both NEEDED this trip. I prayed and stayed pretty calm the first 24-hours, but I didn't unpack, and I didn't even go out on the balcony. How could I go out and look at that beautiful ocean calling my name, if I couldn't stay?

The second day was terrible and Jeff was beside himself. He told me to go down to the beach, but I made the decision if we weren't going to stay, then I didn't want to even see the beach. Moment by moment, a defeated feeling settled in my heart. I was tired, he was mad, and this was not what I had envisioned. The only people I told to pray were my two daughters, so Ellen and Mary Lee were mightily praying.

The morning of day three was the worst, and I'm embarrassed to say--I snapped. Jeff had gotten up, read

his *Jesus Calling,* and as he left to go get a fountain drink at
the store, he said, "Hey, read *Jesus Calling* today," then he
walked out the door.

I made my way to the den and picked up my beauti-
ful leather *Jesus Calling* and turned to October 21st. It was a
long passage, but my eyes only focused in on one line in the
middle of the page. Instead of reading the whole context, all
I could comprehend was that it said something about how
the Lord gives and how He takes away.

Like I said, I snapped, and I was mad. Call it what
you want, "the straw that broke that camel's back" or "the
icing on the cake." I yelled, *"What are you saying God? Are
You saying we are going home? Are You saying You give, then You
take away? That me looking forward to this trip was for nothing?"*

What I did next I am ashamed to tell, but it happened. I ripped up my *Jesus Calling.* Pages from this anointed devotional were now all over the den of the condo. It
felt like I had been betrayed by a best friend and I retaliated.
Through the tears and yelling, I had some pretty ugly words
with God. Words I knew I would have to repent for later.
When Jeff walked in the door, he was a little shocked. I was
ready with my bags packed to go home. He thought I had
lost my mind. He was so confused about the *Jesus Calling,*
because He seemed to get something else out of it. He was
encouraged by it and ready to stay and enjoy the rest of the
week.

"I'm not sure what you read, but I'm at peace and we're staying," he said. He changed clothes, put on his swim trunks, and said, "I'm going down to the beach. You need to come too." Fortunately, from where he was standing, the sofa blocked the confetti devotional on the floor. I kept silent and didn't point it out. He grabbed a towel, a beach chair and left. Jeff was not one to sit down and have a "feelings" discussion. Plus, I think he knew the discussion needed to be between me and God.

So there I was. What exactly happened? It was all a blur...except for crystal clear reality of all the pages ripped from the binding of my devotional. I cried and cried. What had I done? As I apologized to God...and to the book...I took the next thirty minutes and gathered all the pages and put them back in date order. It made the book fatter, but it would be OK. Pitiful to look at, but still anointed. Then, it dawned on me...this was like me. 2 Corinthians 4:8-9 says it best,

> "We are pressed on every side by troubles, but we are not crushed. We are perplexed, but not driven to despair. We are hunted down, but never abandoned by God. We get knocked down, but we are not destroyed." (NLT)

I have to admit every morning for the weeks to come, I would pick up my *Jesus Calling* and before I opened to the day's date, I said to the book again, "I'm so sorry." When we do stupid stuff, like rip up a devotional out of anger, God will redeem and use it for His glory, when we repent and give it to Him. Many times for the next couple of months, God would send me someone who felt guilty because they were angry with God. I would share my wonderful wisdom and experience on the subject, and then show the visual aid to back it up. God never wastes a thing. By the way, the rest of the beach trip was wonderful. So much so, I didn't want to pack!

• • • •

On November 9th, Mama called me and said they took Daddy to the emergency room. Come to find out, there was a host of things wrong with him, including heart issues. He stayed in intensive care and for the first three days, he was somewhat unconscious and hooked up to a IV. The fourth day he came around, but still very weak, but of course, he still maintained his silly humor, which in this situation made me very proud of him. He told me, "Jo, I'm just so weak." I said, "Well Daddy, you haven't had any food--they've just had you on an IV for three days." He looked at me and said, "Well Jo, I think it's because yesterday was Veteran's Day and they led me around the town square in my old Air Force uniform." What? Ha! I laughed out loud and my mother just shook her head and said, "How does he think up such silly stuff?"

Daddy had always been the perfect patient when it came to hospitality with the nurses. He would tell them how good of job they were doing, thank them continuously, and tells them how much he appreciated them. On one day, a drop-dead gorgeous student nurse was shadowing one of the nurses for the whole day. Seriously, she was stunning... perfect face, long black hair, model-like. When I walked in, Daddy insisted that I meet her. So I introduced myself and shook her hand. Daddy proceeded to say, under the influence of medication I might add, "Jo, she is so sweet." He then told her, "Now, I have a son too. I wish you could meet him. He is a good-looking guy. Jo, show her a picture of Jed."

Instantly, I had this figured out! For this brief moment Daddy was thinking of Jed as a 25-year-old, and looking all handsome in his old Air Force uniform. I sweetly said to him, in hopes of bringing him back to reality, "Daddy, I don't think she wants to see a picture of a 50-year-old man."

This sweet young nurse laughed slightly and Daddy had a sober look on his face. It dawned on him that Jed was indeed 50-years-old, heavier and married with two children. As I walked out of his room with her I said, "Hey, I will show you a picture of my cat, Solomon, but I will NOT show you a picture of Jed, because that would just be creepy." She sweetly thanked me.

Not only did Daddy make me laugh, Mama tickled me too. She complimented me on my top and I told her I got it at Kohl's. She said, "Well, I can't seem to find anything there…it's all either 'J Leno' or 'Britney Spears.' OK, I knew she meant "J Lo," but I never corrected her.

As I stayed those days at the hospital, I quickly realized Mama was definitely not up to par in her legs. She was using a cane, but walking very slow. She was still going to have to have more rehab and healing time. I think she knew, that I knew, she had a ways to go on recovery, so she made it a point to bring up my Thanksgiving trip. She made it clear that by no means was I cancelling our trip to Ellen's. She's so precious and I knew she just could not live with the possibility of us staying in town. I decided to trust the timing to God, for Him to continue great healing for her legs and now healing Daddy as well. One thing was certain, Ellen, Joe, Mary Lee, and Jeff were praying hard for us to go! I had peace that God would answer our prayers.

Each day Daddy improved, but it seemed like this was aging him by ten more years. As I looked at him in the hospital, the realization of how long he would live would go through my mind. Being thankful with a grateful heart welled up in me, *"Oh Lord, thank you for the summer. I know I didn't do it all right in attitude or actions, but I'm so glad I had*

that unique time with Daddy." As I talked to God, He gave me
some flashbacks of fun moments with Daddy. He also pointed out that after every meal I made, after every night when
I tucked him in bed, and after every urinal I held, Daddy
would say, "Jo, thank you…I appreciate it." I needed that
reminder and for those memories to stay in the forefront of
my mind. To my daddy, I was still his little girl. Each time
I would leave for Murfreesboro for the past four months he
would say, "Jo, be careful." And now, I appreciated that too.

On November 17th Daddy went to Glen Oaks for
rehab, but I knew his rehab would be different from how my
mother viewed rehab. He wouldn't want to practice walking
or doing the occupational therapy. He would instead want
to watch his ballgames. The day they moved him into his
room, I somehow knew he wouldn't be back home. I knew
he was beyond me taking care of him, and he was definitely
past Mama caring for him. He was even past the caregivers
caring for him. Mama knew it too deep down even though
neither one of us mentioned it to each other. My heart hurt
for him. The whole situation made me so sad. I was most
upset that his routine would change. It was now ironic that
what got on my nerves the most; I now wanted him to have
back.

Knowing Daddy was staying at Glen Oaks, and
Mama had caregivers at the house, made it a bit easier to
leave and go to Colorado. As my family had Thanksgiving

together with Ellen and Joe, I thought about Mama being
alone for their Thanksgiving. She assured me she was fine
and she had FOUR Thanksgiving plates brought to the
house. This made me smile and once again praise God for
the family and friends in Shelbyville. I was humbled when
I thought about those individuals who left their families
for a while to drive to Mama's to make sure she was fed on
Thanksgiving. What an amazing gift of love and kindness!

CHAPTER NINE

The Aftermath

The weeks and months that came brought a flood of emotions I did not expect. I remembered the lady I met at church and the moment we shared about caregiving. I remembered wondering why there was such a "lost" look in her eyes. I thought since her father-in-law had passed, she could have just picked up where she had left off, before she moved him into her home. Things would just return to normal. Now I understood why it did not happen that way at all.

Journal Entries

December 18th

*Lord, I do feel like the summer messed me up emotion-
ally. I still feel so lost and confused. I feel like I've lost
my way and my purpose. I'm trying to really pinpoint
what's nagging me spiritually. Mama's accident
happened so fast and my life changed so fast. I feel
like something could happen and there is no warning
or planning. Logically, I know that's just life, but the
little girl in me has pulled away. I just feel strange.
I've got to practice what I teach about thankfulness
and a grateful heart. Help me Lord to feel alive again.
To have emotion again. To not waste a day because
I'm being lazy or idle. Since I don't see or feel purpose
anymore, help me still be purposeful. Lord, help me.
Please don't let me fall from You. Keep me close and
secure in You. Please say something Lord! As I got
silent before Him, in my heart I heard these words,
"Press In – Push...My Ways are not your ways...
My Thoughts are not your thoughts. Persist in My
Word...Unlock your lips to worship."*

December 21st

*I feel like I'm just existing. No goals, no excitement,
no desires. Nothing. I don't like this feeling. I'm*

*feeling too self-absorbed and I don't like that. It's like I
don't even think about prayer or looking at a situation
with the eyes of faith. I feel lazy and idle and not purposeful. Even though I may "feel" this, I KNOW that
You are my God. I know You love me, and You are
my answer. I WILL TRUST YOU! Thank You for
spiritual seasons, and just maybe, I'm about to start a
new season. The best is yet to come. I feel like David
in the Psalms, and I will encourage myself in the Lord.
I love You, Lord.*

• • • •

My brother Jed and his wife, Missy, came home at
Christmas time and visited Daddy at the nursing home.
They could not believe how much he had declined in his
health. Jed told Mama that she had no choice, but to let this
staff of people at Glen Oaks continue to take care of him. He
saw no possible way of daddy ever returning home and that
Mama would never return to her caregiving role. Jeff had
been telling me the same thing, yet it seemed odd how you
tend to continue to see if there are any other options you
have not thought of. Jed and I talked about the situation
with Mama and she knew this was the next step. I wondered if Jed also knew this visit would be the last time he
would see his Daddy.

• • • •

Journal Entries

December 30th

*Lord, I ask You to heal and restore me. I'm paralyzed
in my heart. I feel lost. I need You to help me find my
way back…back to Your Word…back to the Joy of the
Lord…back to loving and encouraging others. Maybe
it's not going back to those things, but moving forward
in them by faith even when I don't feel it. Lord, "by
faith" help me read the Word…"by faith" help me
praise and worship You with joy…"by faith" help me
to intentionally love and encourage others.*

January 2, 2013

*It's a new year. My mind is a fog. What do I do?
Work? Go back to working with the college age group
at church? Where's my place, Lord? Where are You
going to plant me? I feel so unspiritual. I feel numb
and a little sad. There's something not right with me.
It's like I can't move forward with You, Lord. I want
to, but there's this feeling that I can't trust You and
the paths You choose for me. I'm just scared to trust
You with my heart. I'm not even sure what I'm*

*expecting from You. I just feel numb inside. Help me
Lord to either find my way back, or find a new place in
You that I've never been to. This morning the song in
my head was Jared Anderson's chorus, "We will dance
till the chains fall off." So maybe I start there. I will
be honest Lord, I feel like You don't need me or hear
me. I'm not sure how You feel about me…or how I feel
about You.*

January 3rd

*I tried to exercise, but I had no energy. Why Lord do I
just want to sit and let my mind wander? I feel so
paralyzed. I'm in a fog and I can't lift it, God.*

January 4th

*I'm excited to meet with Laurel today. I guess my
hope is You will tell her to tell me something that will
help. Lord, I have no doubt in You or who You are. I
guess I doubt Your goodness and in the power of
prayer. I have a hard time praying and really believing it helps. It's like I feel what happens is going to
happen, because You control it anyway, so why pray
and believe something I might hope for. If You are in
control, then my hopes, dreams, and desires may
conflict with Your will and may even be selfish.
Maybe I'm supposed to get to this place where I trust*

You and just let what happens happen the way You plan it. I do feel like I'm not joyful, that I still could cry at the drop of a hat. Something is really hurting still in me--something deep. I don't know what to do. I feel like if I worship or praise, it's only to feel better and not because it's the right thing to do, which would be out of love for You. Now You've called me to minister to one of the college girls. I know you have emotional healing for her, but can I really pray in faith for her? I don't want to be a fake Christian, although I'm sure at times I have been and just gone through the motions. I want to be authentic, strong, fearless and confident in You. Maybe this is a part of me letting go...letting go of control, pride, boasting, self-sufficiency and self-ambitions. I don't know.

January 5th

Time with Laurel was so good. She gave me Ephesians 2:8 from the Amplified translation, "For it is by free <u>grace</u> (God's unmerited favor) that you are saved (delivered from judgment and made partakers of Christ's salvation) through [your] faith. And this [salvation] is not of yourselves [of your own doing, it came not through your own striving], but it is the gift of God."

I've been walking with the Lord a long time, yet lately
I've been leaving out a critical component in my walk
with Him…grace. It's like I've been doing the faith
part without the grace part. By grace I can have faith,
but without grace it becomes works of faith…which is
very tiring. And I've realized that so much of my walk
with You has been to "feel" good about me. So now
what Lord? Now I can't do a thing. No more works.
I want a real relationship and to understand how to
live in Your grace, then kick in my faith! I'm tired,
numb and existing, so it's up to You. Thank you for
Laurel and her wisdom. Please bless her, Lord.

The scripture that also came to mind this morning was
Jesus saying, "In this world you will have trials, but
be of good cheer, I've overcome the world." So it is
naïve and immature for me to think certain things
won't happen, but there is a peace in knowing that
Your hand is on me and my family.

January 6th

What an amazing Sunday! The worship was so good
today…brought me to tears. I took a nap and when I
woke up my friend, Tracie and Mama had texted me. I
called Mama first. She said Daddy told her that he
didn't think he was going to walk again and thought it

was best he stayed at the nursing home. I'm sure
Mama was shocked. She told him she and I had
discussed it and she wanted him OK with becoming a
resident there. He asked if she would be OK at home
by herself. She assured him she would be fine and that
we would bring his recliner and make the room
comfortable. He also asked if he could NOT do any
more rehab. She told him he would have to do a couple
of days a week just for his health. Mama said the
whole conversation made the guilt lift off her shoul-
ders. She had been feeling guilty thinking it was her
fault Daddy was in the nursing home, or at least it
sped up the process of him being there. She was so
scared he would resent her. I believe God prepared
Daddy's heart and gave him peace in knowing this was
his new residence. I'm sure when all of this sinks in,
Mama will shed some tears, but God, I know now You
have been there the whole time. You have prepared the
way. You will carry Mama through and You will comfort her through this transition. And God...take care
of Daddy. I underestimated You and I underestimated
him. However long his days are on earth, let them be
good. Thank You.

The next text from Tracie was about a song her
preacher talked about during his sermon. It was

BLESSINGS by Laura Story. The words are amazing and oh so true. As I listened to the song on my computer, it brought so much encouragement. God, I'm living Romans 8:28 - "ALL things DO work together for good for those who are IN Christ Jesus." God, I don't know what to say but "THANK YOU." If it is Your plan and by Your grace, I'd like to write a book.

January 30th

Lord, I haven't journaled in a while. I try to go see Daddy twice a week. His room is nice and across the hall from his old friend, Whitey. Daddy decided no more therapy because all it did was just make him mad. All the pep talks from Mama and all her trying to logically explain the benefits of rehab didn't do a bit of good. I told Mama, "He's 83-years-old, therefore he gets to choose. Even if you think it's a wrong choice, take what he loves and focus on that...food, baths, ballgames and naps."

Over the last three days Daddy has been really sick. When I saw him Monday his eyes looked so weak, but he still had a sense of humor...just a weak delivery. The doctor told Mama he had pneumonia. Today he's on breathing treatments, but he's still throwing up.

Lord, I had an unsettling feeling. Daddy says all the time, "I'm just tired." He even asked Mama, "What did I do to deserve this?" This hurts my heart. Today I can't stop tearing up. Are You taking him soon, Lord? I don't want him to go sad or thinking You are unfair or cruel. I know You are a good God, but I guess life is just unfair and sometimes very cruel. Can I make a request? Before it is time for him to go with You, will You flood him with peace and give him a vision of his friends (who have already passed) standing with Jesus, all happy and excited to see him.

January 31st

Coffee with my dear friend, Shelly, is always a special blessing. She is my "princess warrior" because she pushes, challenges, and refreshes my soul with the truth of God's Word. In talking with her I realized some feelings surfaced. One, that I'm cool with Jesus and the Holy Spirit. It's like I feel they are "for me." But I'm heavy at times talking with God, trusting Him and seeing Him as loving and good. I know I can't separate the Trinity, but this distinct feeling I could pinpoint. I wonder will He really do miracles for me (yet I know He truly does). I also feel like this summer I was "benched from the game." I've always been active in my faith and in the Body of Christ...out

there in the field, but it feels like He has pulled me
from the game and stuck me right on the bench. When
I see that vision, I can clearly see Jesus and the Holy
Spirit on the bench with me, so it is not a bad place to
be. Maybe He pulled me from the game because I
sometimes dominate the field. Shelly said as I teach
others the Word, maybe I need more God perspective
and for me to let God be bigger than me. That I should
allow Him to control more, stretch me more, and for
me to trust Him more. She believed this was an area of
pride that God so graciously wants to realign me in. I
truly want to cooperate with Him and let Him do His
work in me and while I'm on the bench, I want to be a
worshipper there. Lord, help me trust You and allow
You to be the "Coach" in my life.

February 2nd (1:47 am)

I've been awake thinking about Mary Lee and school,
then suddenly the Lord gave me a vision. I could see
Daddy laying in the nursing home bed and how sad I
was watching him. I asked the Lord, "Has he asked
You to come take him home?" The Lord said, "Yes."
Then I saw myself walking in Daddy's room. He was
lying on his back with his mouth open, trying to
breathe. I bent down and kissed his forehead. Jesus
was standing on the other side of the bed. Jesus

*extended His right hand and grabbed daddy's hand.
Immediately, Daddy woke up and looked at Jesus.
Jesus helped him out of the bed and Daddy suddenly
looked 20 years younger. He grabbed Jesus' shoulder
and patted Him on the back and said in the most
sincere way, "Thank You...I appreciate it." Daddy
looked at me, smiled and winked. It was brief because
he was so excited to be leaving with Jesus. When they
left the room, Daddy had on his dress shirt and pressed
khaki dress pants...and he was walking just fine. As
they walked out of the room door, the scene switched to
heaven. All of Daddy's friends were waiting for him.
The reunion was like little boys laughing, cutting-up
and playing. Jesus was happy. I looked back at the bed
in the nursing home...it was empty.*

February 4th

*Well the second burden was lifted from Mama today.
She called me this afternoon and said Daddy was
sitting in his chair and he motioned for her to come
over. Since he had lost his voice from the pneumonia,
he had to still whisper. She bent down and he said,
"Mama, I want to tell you how proud I am of how well
you've done with your legs." Mama had still been
carrying the guilt of having the accident, thinking
again, it contributed to him being in the nursing home*

faster. Logically she knew it wasn't true, but the feelings were still there. She was a little in shock by his statement. She said, "Well, I've just done what they have told me to do. During these cold days, it has been hard, but I keep trying." She told me what she really wanted to do was burst into tears and have a good cry. God, You are so amazing. Thank You for lifting this off of Mama and please bless Daddy for humbling himself to bless her.

CHAPTER TEN

The Lord Prepares

D addy lived at the nursing home for six months. Mama did everything she could to make his room look homey. She put up photographs of all of his immediate family, including my cat Solomon. Daddy was always a cat lover, so that particular picture made him smile. She brought from home side tables and a lamp to dress up the room. She also took devotionals that she read to him daily.

Even though Daddy seemed to recover from the pneumonia, he continued to get weaker and more feeble. It was ironic to see the difference in Mama and Daddy. Mama

was improving by leaps and bounds, and Daddy was declining also with those same jumps. Physically, he could not
walk anymore. His legs were like toothpicks and his feet
stayed numb due to little circulation. From his waist down,
he was almost paralyzed.

Mentally, he also continued to decline. I don't know
if it was from the dementia or just a natural deterioration
with age, but he had a hard time processing the simplest of
things. It was as if words were confusing and jumbled up
when he would hear them. At first, we thought the problem
was his hearing aid, then he admitted to Mama that he could
hear fine, but her words were hard to understand. Mama
would ask him simple questions like, "Billy, do you want
the television on or off?" He would just stare at her a second
then say, "Mama, please don't ask me questions." Some
days he would get so irritated with her for no reason. She
didn't let it bother her because she understood that he just
didn't feel good.

Most of the time, Daddy stayed very hospitable to
the nurses. He told them frequently how much he appreciated them, whether they came in with medicine, changed his
clothes, or just brought his meals. They loved Daddy and
tried to please him and make him comfortable and peaceful.
Some of the nurses adored him so much that they would kiss
him on the forehead or pat the top of his head. Even when
he was sharp-tongued with them, he always apologized and

asked for their forgiveness. Well, that just made them love him more!

One thing that stayed intact most of the time was Daddy's appetite. That man could always eat! Since the nursing home gave him insulin for his diabetes, he pretty much ate what he wanted. Mama would bring food from home, like meatloaf or spaghetti, and he would be so excited. Even though the nursing home food was good, his wife's home-cooking couldn't be beat in Daddy's eyes. He would first eat what she brought him, and then when the nurse would come in with his lunch, he would eat that too!

I continued to visit a couple of times a week and surprise him with burgers, reuben sandwiches, KFC, loaded salads or milkshakes. When I would walk in the door of his room I would just stop and pause in front of him. He would focus in on me, then smile and say, "Jo, I'm glad to see you...what did you bring me?" Then he would follow up by saying, "Jo, I don't want you to feel like you have to always bring me something...but I appreciate it when you do." I remembered those months of dreading all of the cooking and being frustrated with the rotations of meals. Now, I wanted to please him and bring him treats to make his day.

Mama's healing and recovery was nothing short of amazing. For the six months Daddy was in the nursing home, Mama had the routine of waking up about 9:00 am, rehabbing and exercising her legs for an hour at home, and

then she would get dressed to drive to see Daddy at 11:00
am, staying with him till about 2:00 pm. Just as he was used
to going to bed at home at 9:00 pm sharp, he was ready
to take his nap at 2:00 pm sharp. He would even watch
the clock on the wall and as it was approaching naptime,
he would tell Mama to help him get into bed. In the six-
months time period, Mama only missed three days of not
going to the nursing home. Two of those days were due
to bad weather and the other was for her doctor's appointment. I admired her faithfulness so much, and no doubt the
nurses always looked forward to seeing her. When those
nurses took care of her just a few months earlier, she was
in a wheelchair and couldn't walk. Seeing her walk up and
down the halls was very cool to them and made them proud.
Mama became so strong and improved in her walking, that
by the first of the year she started staying at home by herself.
Thus ended the role of the outside caregivers and Mama officially had her house back.

  Since her house had been "Daddy-proofed" over the
years because he used a walker, she moved around furniture, unrolled rugs and set coffee tables out. The house
looked great. Mama and Daddy married when she was
17-years-old, so it dawned on me that this was the first time
in her whole life she had ever lived by herself. It was also
the first time in years she only had to take care of herself.
She could get up when she wanted to, go to bed when she

wanted to, and there was no one beckoning her…for anything. Did you know it's OK to miss someone with all your
heart, yet feel freedom at the same time? Did you know it's
OK to enjoy spending time with someone, yet enjoy quiet
time alone? It is OK, because God is in both.

As springtime came and the cold weather was leaving, Daddy started asking Mama if he could get out some.
What he desired and brought to her attention often was how
much he wanted to eat at Legends, a nice steakhouse restaurant. He and I ate there a couple of times a month for special
outings when Mama was in the nursing home. Mama told
him she would take him, but they had to wait for a warm
day. She consulted with me to help decide if this was a good
idea. I thought it was, but we would have to do it together.
Since he was scheduled to have a doctor's appointment in
early April, we decided this would be the perfect day to ven-
ture out and have lunch.

When the special day arrived, one of the nurses
helped us load him in the car. Unfortunately, it did not take
long for us to realize this was not going to be easy. Compared to when I use to take him to see Mama in the nursing
home, he was like night and day. In just a few months he
had declined to where he couldn't stand, and mentally he
was in a fog. When I tried to help him go from the car to the
wheelchair, he almost landed in the parking lot. He seemed
to panic and go limp, so I was picking him up with all my

strength. I felt a little panicked too, thinking if he missed the transfer from seat to seat and he fell, he would have broken some bones. With every transfer, he was more and more scared and weak. We made it to the restaurant, but it wasn't a pretty sight. It was as if he had lost his motor skills. Food was landing in his lap and when people would speak to him he seemed confused. This man was the social champion of Shelbyville, and now he was oblivious to other people. It was just pitiful and I was heartbroken. I was sitting across from my daddy, who was so different just nine months earlier. By the time we got back to the nursing home he was exhausted...and so were we. He quickly said, "I don't think I want to do that anymore." I was glad he came to that conclusion, because the whole outing was dangerous.

At the end of April, he had totally forgotten the outing and decided he wanted to try and get out again. This time he just wanted Mama to ride him around town, but let him stay in the car. I offered to come and help, but she said a couple of the nurses would get him in the car and out of the car when they returned, so all she had to do was chauffer.

Later that day I called Mama to see how the ride went. She said, "Honey, he hardly acknowledged anything. I even drove him by the house and he didn't even look over. When I tried to make conversation and point out things, he finally said, 'Rhoda, whew...please...you're making me nervous.' I asked him if he just wanted to be quiet and he said 'yes.'" I am not sure how much he enjoyed the outing, but one thing was for certain...it wore him out...and it would be his last outing.

For the six months at Glen Oaks, he never once asked about going home or about the house in general. He didn't even ask how long he had been there. It was like he just knew this was where he was supposed to be. All he wanted to know was whether Mama would be back the next day. He looked forward to seeing her and would tell her, "It just gets so lonely. Mama, I don't know what I would do if you didn't come."

On the days I didn't go see Daddy, I would always call Mama to see how he was doing. We talked about how we didn't like him living in a nursing home, but we knew Mama could not take care of him anymore. In fact, even the caregivers couldn't take care of him anymore. This was the next phase, even though it was sad. In a phone conversation one day Mama shared with a heavy heart and said, "I just feel so bad, because I always told your daddy I would take care of him as long as I could."

I assured her by saying, "But Mama....you did! You kept your word...you kept him as long as you possibly could." I knew and she knew deep down that if the accident had not happened, the time of her being sole-caregiver was quickly coming to an end. Her friends would tell her frequently, "Rhoda, you are wearing yourself out! This is not healthy for you. You are spoiling him, and you are jeopardizing your own health." None the less, she was determined to take care of him as long as she was physically able. She just did not expect it to ever really come to an end. She did not expect the decision to be made for her, but that she would decide the time-frame of when being his caregiver was over. I understood how she felt, except I did not control when I was called and she did not control when she was dismissed. In both cases, your life changes suddenly, therefore, you have to dig deep in your faith and hang on to the only One who is totally in control...Jesus.

• • • •

Toward the end of April, Joe and Ellen came for a visit from Colorado Springs. On Sunday after church, my whole family drove over in two cars to see Daddy. Ellen and I had already had the conversation that this would probably be the last time she would see her Papa BI. Daddy seemed tired as we visited that day. He tried to cut-up and be funny, but it was difficult. He was just so weak and too many people in the room made him nervous. Yet, he graciously said to Jeff, "You and Jo sure do have a good-looking family." Jeff would say back, "Well, you started it!" He smiled.

Before we left, the girls wanted their picture made with Daddy. He enjoyed that and was so proud of them.

As they all said their goodbyes and kissed and hugged their papa, a sadness seemed to hit them all, especially Ellen. As we walked out the doors of the nursing home, Ellen headed straight for the car. I watched her get in and break-down in tears. I knew and she knew she wouldn't see him again.

• • • •

Daddy turned 84-years-old on May 21st. I took him one of his favorite meals from a restaurant in Murfreesboro and drove over to visit him. I also decided to write in his birthday card the vision the Lord gave me about Jesus coming to get him one day and all of his friends in heaven waiting on him. Even though Daddy was a believer, I didn't know how he really felt about death and dying. I just didn't want him scared or worried, so maybe the card would help him look forward to his eternal home and he would know he was not alone in the journey. When I arrived with the food, he was very pleased. He didn't do a lot of talking, just eating.

Later in the afternoon I received a text from Mama that said she read the birthday card to Daddy and they both had cried with joyful tears. *"Lord, I pray the vision brings him continued peace and anticipation in the days to come."*

• • • •

On Tuesday, May 28th, I met Mama at the nursing home for a regular visit. When it was time for Daddy's nap, she tucked him in and we both kissed him bye. As always he would tell me, "I love you Jo and I always look forward to seeing you." Each time he would tell me his voice was weaker, but those words became sweeter and sweeter to hear. I knew he really meant it, and I looked forward to seeing him too.

Instead of going back to Murfreesboro, I asked Mama if I could come over and visit. At her house we relaxed for a while and just talked about Daddy, the girls, and general small talk. When it was time to head home, I thought about Daddy again. As I was leaving Shelbyville the Lord spoke in my heart, *"Go back by the nursing home."* I turned on a side road and drove straight there. I knew there was a purpose, but I didn't want to ask the Lord why. I would just go back, no questions asked.

When I walked by the nurse's station, one of them said, "What are you doing back?" I kept walking, smiled and said, "Forgot something!"

I knew Daddy would be asleep and without his hearing aid, he would not hear a thing. As I walked in the door, I saw him laying there like a little boy all curled up on

his side. I took a couple of steps toward him and he started
jerking a little, like he was restless. I took steps back towards
the door and just squatted down. If he happened to open his
eyes, I didn't want to scare him.

"*Lord, I'm not sure what to do. I'll just pray.*" I softly
prayed for him, for his peace and for God to help him. I
thanked God for his life and for letting him be my daddy. I
thanked God for the months we were together and for letting
me care for him. Then, I just thanked and praised God for
being so good.

After about ten minutes I left and drove back to Murfreesboro. "*Is it soon God? Jesus, will You be getting him soon?*"

• • • •

The next day, on Wednesday, May 29th, Mama went
at her normal time to see Daddy. He picked at his lunch and
seemed to be very agitated. Mama sensed he was unusually
uncomfortable, so she asked one of the nurses to check his
vitals. Well, this made him more agitated. He sternly said,
"I just want to be left alone." As the nurses would ask him
questions, he continued to say more forcefully, "I just want
to be left alone!" Finally, Mama cued the nurses to leave and
she helped Daddy into bed for his nap. She kissed him bye,
but was unsettled to leave him in this condition, yet he kept
telling her he wanted to be left alone.

At 10:30 pm that night her phone rang. She knew it

was the nursing home before she answered. "Mrs. Gunter…
Mr. Gunter is being taken to the Emergency Room. His
doctor wants him to go." Mama told them she would meet
them there. When she texted me to let me know, I remembered my extra visit the day before. *"Oh Lord, this quick? Are
you coming for him tonight?"*

Mama said she would call me when she got to the
hospital, but I told Jeff we had better change clothes and
head to Shelbyville. Mary Lee got up and knew she better
go too. As we got in the car, Mama texted again to say we
had better come on quickly.

The drive seemed as long as it did on June 6th when
I drove to the ER for Mama. Mary Lee was in the backseat
with her arm stretched out so her sweet hand rested on my
shoulder. We rode in silence as I kept my cell phone in my
hand anticipating the next text. About ten miles from the
hospital my cell went off. I held my breath as I read the text
from Mama:

"He passed. I'll call Jed." – 11:24pm

My cry came out of my mouth before my thoughts
understood the words of the text. Mary Lee kept her hand
on me, as she softly sobbed from the backseat. Jeff reached
over and tightly held my hand. *"My daddy died, oh My Lord,
my daddy has died"*, was all I could think of.

As we pulled into the parking lot, Jeff had barely put
the car in park before I jumped out and sprinted towards the

ER. As soon as the admitting staff person saw me, she hit
the button to open the double doors. As I ran down the hall,
I saw a few nurses gathered outside a curtain-closed room. I
knew Daddy was there. When I walked around the curtain,
there stood Mama and there laid Daddy. He looked just
like I remembered in my vision when Jesus came to get him.
Mama walked over and we hugged tightly. She quietly said,
"Honey, he's gone."

The ER doctor said he had a very hard heart attack
and went quickly. I walked over to him and touched his
forehead. It was cold…a cold shell. My Jesus did what He
said. He took him home. I felt sadness and I felt joy. God
is in both. Daddy was in heaven with his friends. He was
home and he was free.

We stood there for a while, just looking at Daddy. I
looked at Mary Lee and her sweet face was so sad. She had
lost her first grandparent. Even though she was hurting, I
was so glad she was there. This may sound strange, but seeing my husband shed tears for my daddy was such a blessing. Jeff loved my daddy very much. He respected him, enjoyed visiting him and most of all, he thought my daddy was
one of the most hilarious men he had ever met. Daddy had
made Jeff laugh so many times over years. What a blessing
to know he would miss him as much as I would.

As we left the Emergency Room, I told Mama I
would stay with her for the night. She didn't argue at all.

By the time we got to the house it was about 12:30 am. I was exhausted, but somehow just could not sleep. Mama was wide awake, so as soon as we changed clothes, she proceeded to get out a legal pad and write down who she needed to call when the sun came up. She pulled out her prepared funeral arrangements and discussed each item with me. Mama was true to her efficient nature, yet not at all insensitive. She cried and said, "Honey, I still can't believe he's gone." Then we would get tickled at something funny Daddy would say, knowing our fatigue was actually helping the situation. Finally, at 3:00 am, she decided we better try to sleep. I could not hold my eyes open any longer. I had about three hours of sleep, but Mama never closed her eyes. I knew she wasn't alone though. I knew my Jesus was near and His Spirit was comforting her. He draws near to the brokenhearted, so I knew she was in good hands.

• • • •

Just as Mama had all of their finances organized, she also had burial details as well. There was no questions or surprises, because she had it all planned out over the years. When I met her at the funeral home to go over details, I was expecting the director and pastor to do most of the talking and ask the questions making it about a two to three hour process. Well, true to her gifts and talents, just like Donald Trump, my mother sat down and conducted the discussion

like a board meeting. She had her binder and list of questions, so the whole thing took less than thirty minutes. I
think the funeral director and Brother Tom was impressed
and very pleased that the time together was efficient and
well thought out. I came home that day and told Jeff how
proud I was of Mama. In the midst of heartache and loss,
she had the ability to move forward with grace and style.

We decided to have the visitation and funeral all
in the same day, both at First Christian Church on a Sunday afternoon. On June 2nd as the time of visitation ap-
proached, friends and family flooded in the church. For the
three hours of visitation, people were wrapped around the
church waiting to share their condolences with our family. I
thought about the spiritual law of "sowing and reaping" and
all the years Daddy sowed into going to other's visitations.
I remembered how he would bring the gift of memories
and stories to the grieving families to bless them and bring
a smile to their face. Now he was reaping. By the time the
funeral service began, the sanctuary was full.

Mama had asked me to give the eulogy, which I was
honored to do. I have never really had a fear of speaking in
front of people, but this was a little different. I was used to
teaching bible studies, and speaking in front of women's or
college groups, so I had to really pray about how this was
going to go. My thoughts went to my funny Daddy and
if he was sitting on the front row, how would he want his

eulogy delivered. No doubt, it had to be light-hearted and maybe even times of laughter. Sad moments made him uncomfortable. Since Daddy had the ability to lighten-up the atmosphere, I would make that my goal. I wanted to make him proud and make him smile.

When it was my turn to speak, I took a deep breath and walked up the steps to the podium. I decided to take a second and look at the people. It was a beautiful sight. I spotted my friend, Kelly Rollins. I instantly remembered he had spoken at two family funerals himself, so without thinking, the first words out of my mouth were, "Pray for me Kelly." He knew what I was feeling for sure. In my heart I asked the Holy Spirit to be Lord over my words, gestures and emotions. I wanted this moment to bless my daddy's memory, to bless this room of special, loving people, but most of all, I wanted to please my Lord. This was the actual eulogy:

First of all, thank you for coming today. But more than that, thank you for the way you have served, prayed and loved our family over the last several years, especially over this past year. Mama and Daddy have been blessed with the most awesome, generous and loving friends. And no doubt Jeff and I have been abundantly blessed in this area as well. There is nothing like the Body of Christ. I truly believe that one of the most amazing ideas God had was to use the people of God to encourage and serve one another in His Name, and this community has done that beautifully. On behalf of our family, Thank You.

Billy Gunter. Just saying his name brings a smile, doesn't it? He was a very unique man. As my mother would say, "There's not a serious bone in your father's body." When our family needed a "straight man," Mama had to play that role, because Daddy couldn't do it. Daddy just couldn't be serious, even in serious circumstances. For example, In 1994 Daddy had bypass surgery and while he was in the hospital they decided to also do a prostate procedure, and found fluid on the brain requiring a shunt. Poor Jed was in Arizona and called Daddy and said, "Daddy, what's going on? First it was just bypass, and then I hear there doing this and then that…Do I need to come? I just don't understand what's going on?" Daddy calmly said, "Well son, they were running this special."

I can also remember Mama sharing with me when they were rolling daddy in for surgery and he's lying on the gurney and my precious mother leans over his face and compassionately says, "Now Honey, they are taking you for surgery. You're going to be alright, and I'm going to be right here when you get back." Daddy says back, "Mama, you need a mint." Just couldn't be serious.

Last November when Daddy was in intensive care, the first three days he was out of it and on an IV. The fourth day he came around, yet he was still so weak. But of course, he still maintained his silly humor, which I have to admit made me very proud of him. He told me, "Jo, I'm just so weak." I said, "Well Daddy, you haven't had any food…they've just had you on IV's for three days."

He looked at me and said, "Well Jo, I think it's because yesterday was Veteran's Day and they led me around the town square in my old Air Force uniform." I laughed out loud and my mother just shook her head and said, "How does he think up such stuff?"

Daddy had the gift of silly. He was the master at having a good laugh and producing laughter in others. If I wrote down all of the little sayings and silly remarks my daddy used to say, there wouldn't be a large enough book to contain them. And what good are silly remarks but to be passed down, so I'm sure Jed would agree that we catch ourselves saying them, thinking them or sharing them quite a bit. Jeff and I have been married for 28 years and to this day, I'll think of something and say to Jeff, "Hey you know what Daddy use to say?" Jeff would be all ears because he knew he was going to laugh...sometimes till he cried. Daddy also had word triggers, which was a word that would remind him of another word. For example, this past summer when I was living with Daddy, we would go thru the same silly routines every day... just for the sake of keeping the atmosphere light. Daddy had a shaving routine in the mornings. He would be sitting in the den chair watching <u>The Price is Right</u> and say, "Jo, while I'm sitting here I'll shave, so hand me my razor...Joe Frazier." Every single morning for three months, he would say, "Jo hand me my razor"... and my line was... Joe Frazier. I even called Mama while she was rehabbing at Glen Oaks and asked, "If I said get me my razor, what would you say?" And she said, "Joe Frazier."

While I lived with Daddy last summer, one night he re-

quested soup for supper. He always ate a light supper anyway, so
I thought soup would be great sense it was quick and easy. Now
this was my kind of cooking! Well, "easy to fix" backfired on me.
Daddy was up that night at 11:30, 2:15, 5:15 and 6:30. He felt so
bad after the first three times, because I was up holding the urinal. Each time he would say, "Jo, I'm so sorry. I shouldn't have
eaten soup." I would say, "It's OK, Daddy." And he would just
shake his head, like he was disgusted at himself. But at 6:30 am as
we stood together and he was going in the urinal he said, "Jo, I've
decided I want soup for breakfast." With his hearing aid out, he
couldn't even hear me laugh. I was exhausted, but that was hilarious.

Daddy was a story teller. I have had so many people tell me
over the years, "I love to hear your daddy tell a story." Daddy had
an amazing memory, so when he told a story it was with all the
details. Actually, sometimes he would "brighten" the details, but
only for the sake of the entertainment of the story. Mama, Jed and
I have heard the same stories over and over and over, but honestly,
they remained funny. I can also say living with him last summer
and hearing them, those stories became much sweeter to my heart.

Daddy was an ambassador. What I mean was Daddy loved to
socialize and introduce people to other people. He loved to socially
work a funeral. Because of his memory he could share a story
about the loved one and the family would smile, sometimes even
laugh. The grocery store was probably where he socialized the
most. Daddy always did the grocery shopping and loved it. Grow-

ing up I can remember him leaving about 8:00 or 9:00 on Saturday mornings and sometimes wouldn't get back until noon. This was not because of a long grocery list, but he was busy talking, laughing and meeting new people in the community. When Jeff and I got married I think we even discussed sending a wedding invitation to the grocery store. Speaking of our wedding, I remember walking down the aisle with Daddy and he waved back and forth at everyone. Funny, I thought the day was about me! :)

When I think about what my daddy loved the most were people. It didn't matter a person's race, age, or background. He appreciated people and he loved to tell you that he appreciated you. When we would be at a restaurant, he would always grab the waiter or waitress' arm when they brought something, like ketchup, and he would say, "Thank you, I appreciate it." I'm sure the Glen Oaks nurses would tell you he told them many times, "Thank you, I appreciate your help." And by the way, God bless the staff at Glen Oaks. You guys were the hands and feet of Christ and please know that we DO appreciate you.

Daddy loved First Christian Church and his church family. And he dearly loved the children in the church. Up until Daddy was homebound, he was always at church on Sunday. Growing up, Daddy loved dressing up for church. On Sunday mornings he would have on his jacket and tie, then make his way to Jed's room to find his baseball bat. He'd pick it up and say, "Jed, I better take this to knock all the women off." Mama would just shake her head. Jed and I thought it was funny every time. He also loved hearing

sermons at church...although there was that one time my mother
told me, "Well at church today your father cleaned out his wallet."

Daddy loved and appreciated his children. He was a good
Daddy to me and Jed. He was proud of us. He was proud to
introduce us to people and from what I understand over the years
while he was at the Post Office, he showed our pictures to many
people. He was proud of his grandchildren. Of course, when any
of them would tell him about the good grades they made in school,
Daddy's line was always the same, "Well now, you get that from
your papa." He appreciated his sister, Mary Ann. My favorite
thing about their relationship was her calling him brother. He was
a good brother and he would always say, "Mary Ann's the best."
And to Laura (Mary Ann's daughter), he loved you so much. He
was proud to have walked you down the aisle at your wedding. He
was so proud of your boys...mainly because they would always
hug their Uncle Billy.

Most of all he appreciated and loved his wife. I know she's my
mother, but Rhoda Gunter is a faithful wife. As her friends would
agree, she babied Daddy... and I love that. Over the last several
years of being his caregiver, it wasn't easy, but my mother contin-
ued to do an exceptional, selfless job taking care of Daddy. I re-
member when I took Daddy to Glen Oaks to see Mama for the first
time after her accident. She felt so bad, yet was anxious to see him.
As I rolled him over to her bed, He leaned over from his wheelchair
and the first words he said were, "You're tough as nails and you'll
be back." OK, that wasn't the most romantic thing to say, but for

Daddy I knew it was a high compliment and the kind of person he knew she was. He was right. Most 25-year-olds could not have recovered the way she has. Daddy spent the last six months at Glen Oaks and for the exception of 3 days due to the weather; Mama went to the nursing home everyday to continue taking care of him. Tomorrow is their 57th wedding anniversary. I know if Daddy were here he would say, "Mama, you are an amazing woman. Thank you, I appreciate all you've done."

As Daddy's health declined these last few months, Mama and Daddy would discuss details of their final wishes. One day Mama asked him, "Now Billy, listen to me… out of these pictures which one do you want at the funeral?" He glanced over them then said, "Surprise me." :)

Life was becoming very tiring for Daddy. He would tell me and Mama, "I'm so tired." We knew he was so ready, yet death can come so quickly. But there's one thing I know beyond a shadow of a doubt…Wednesday night, Jesus came to see Daddy. He walked over, touched his shoulder and Daddy got up. As I close my eyes, I can see him in his pressed pants and dress shirt. While he grabbed Jesus by the arm, he pats Him on the shoulder and says, "Thank you, I appreciate it."

Proverbs 17:22 says, "A cheerful heart is good medicine."

I think when we all think about Billy Gunter; we will smile and have cheerful memories, maybe even laugh. Because that would make HIM smile.

We love you, Daddy :)

When I sat down I knew Daddy was smiling and saying, "Jo, that was good." Mama and my brother, Jed, approved of the eulogy which made me also smile. *"Thank you Lord for this opportunity to honor my daddy in the way he would have loved it."*

• • • •

It's been a couple of months since Daddy passed. It's been over a year since Mama's accident. Time is a funny thing. It does go by so quickly. I have often thought about the lessons I learned from taking care of Daddy and Mama. Most definitely my faith grew and my compassion for other caregivers developed. God taught me more about humility and how to persevere, and even when I felt like I was exhausted and worn out, there was always more I could give. I knew the scripture was true and "I can do all things through Him who gives me strength."(Philippians 4:13) I knew God would call on me again one day to take care of Mama. Of course, she may be 100-years-old by the time she needs any assistance! I learned so much from God through the lives of my parents.

Daddy taught me to never go through a day without having a good laugh. He taught me to always let people know how much you appreciate them, especially when they are serving. He taught me sharing good stories keeps memories alive and can bring smiles to listening faces. He also taught me that variety in life is important...especially with food!

Mama taught me how to never give up and to keep moving forward. She taught me determination, discipline and endurance. She taught me that no matter how bad things look, you can always be thankful and positive. She taught me that heroes are underestimated and sometimes overlooked, so when you find one, Praise God for them. Praise God for my mother, Rhoda Gunter...she is my hero.

Above all else, God taught me how to start trusting Him more (Proverbs 3:5-6). He is such a big God and He is so aware of each of us. Life can be so difficult at times, as He told us it would be (John 16:33), yet He promises never to leave us, nor forsake us (Hebrews 13:5b). He promises to work ALL things out for good for those who love Him (Romans 8:28). He is such an amazing God and I love Him so.

To all of the caregivers out there who cook, clean, hold urinals, and do countless things that I never even did... you are my heroes too, especially the ones I don't even know. Psalm 16:3 says, *"The godly people in the land are my true heroes! I take pleasure in them!"* I believe it is OK to insert your name in this scripture, or I'll just call you "caregiver." So the scriptures would read:

"The caregivers in the land are my true heroes! I take pleasure in them!"

May God Bless Your Caregiving Days, Keep You Filled and Restore You...Body, Soul and Spirit!

Epilogue

After Daddy passed, Mama had another right leg surgery to remove all of the hardware. This helped with some of the pain from the accident, but it did not change the arthritis in her knee. The "bone on bone" was getting worse and worse, so she finally agreed that it was time for knee replacement. In April 2014, she had the surgery and decided to spend her two weeks of rehab back at Glen Oaks. The staff was excited to see her and true to her character, she rehabbed like a pro. Afterwards, she went home and was able to have her ole pal, PT Mike, back for home therapy.

Jeff bought me a bird feeder and purchased birdfeed
that draws the redbirds--and it certainly did!!! I love to go
out on my back porch in the early morning and watch the
birds. As beautiful as the male redbirds are, I have come
to appreciate the females. They don't have the bright red
feathers, but as my daughter Ellen says, they have on their
red lipstick! There is a lot of symbolism in this when I think
of the bright and colorful personality of my daddy, and the
strong, subtle, persevering personality of my mother. She
definitely wears red lipstick very well.

I haven't returned to a full-time job, but I know God
is leading me to my next assignment soon. I continue to
teach and mentor the college age at church, which blesses
me beyond measure. They keep me young, and I equally
learn so much from them.

Although I don't drive to Shelbyville every day, I
do talk to Mama on the phone almost daily. The faithful
Shelbyville friends and neighbors still act like the beautiful
Body of Christ and are always checking on mama. Because
of her servant's heart, Mama stays busy being a blessing to
others by taking food here and there to the friends in need.
What an amazing cycle of giving and loving!

I think about Daddy often. In a few weeks it will be
one year since he went home to Jesus. My, my...time is a
funny thing. I reflect back on our time together and smile a
lot. I also catch myself thinking about little girl times with

him. The times when he would take me to the public swim-
ming pool, and actually get in the water and swim with
me and my friends. The times when I would go to the post
office while he was working, and he would walk me around
so I could visit all his co-worker buddies. The times when
we would never miss an episode of *Sonny and Cher*, *Tom
Jones*, or *Columbo*. Even though I have just turned fifty, I feel
like a little girl thinking of these memories…the sights, the
feelings, the smells, and the laughter. They make me proud
to be Billy Gunter's daughter. On a bigger scale, I think
somewhat that same way when I think about my Heavenly
Father. He likes me to be "little" with Him. He likes when
I imagine crawling up in His arms and enjoying just being
with Him. He likes me being child-like with Him because
I have more faith and trust in this place. I'm so proud to be
His daughter and that He is proud of me…no matter what.

When I pray for others who are taking care of parents, it seems to have taken on a new meaning. I talk to
friends and hear their stories of caregiving which humble
me. Day after day, year after year, they do the job with the
strength of the Lord. No matter what degree of difficulty
and no matter the length of time their caregiving story tells,
God is faithful. As they share how they gave their anger,
hurt, fatigue, frustration, and disappoint to God, He gives
them in return His amazing peace, contentment, refreshment, joy and hope. There has to be an exchange. When

we lay down those things that weigh us down, and are too heavy for our emotions to carry...yes, when we lay them at His feet, THEN we have to ask Him to give us something in return. We wait and receive from Him. He is such a good gift giver. He'll even send redbirds.

Hidden Crosses Paintings

In seeing God's hand in many areas of my life, I began painting abstracts and hiding crosses in the painting. This signified the personal trials we all go through, yet when we yield to God; He is present and will reveal His unending faithfulness. In fact, as we grow in our relationship with God, we realize the profound reality that God is always in our lives, yet during difficult times, we sometimes aren't aware of His presence.

My newest Hidden Crosses Paintings line shows the Crosses more vibrant and apparent, signifying 2017 is a season of being a bold witness in living out our Christian walk. Each of my paintings is "One of a Kind - Prayed Over and Blessed." I desire for each one to be an expression of God's amazing love for us.

The Cross of Jesus Christ is powerful. Through the Cross, there is forgiveness, healing, restoration, redemption, salvation, and well, EVERYTHING you need.

Hidden Crosses Paintings represent places in our lives God has touched, but it is not apparent at the time. Later, as we seek Him and REALLY look, it is obvious where He has been!

For more information and art dealer locations, visit hiddencrosses.com

Blessings!

Mary Jo Graham

Psalm 9:1-2

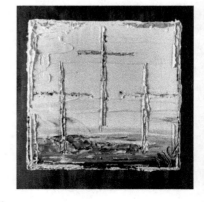

234